IVF DIET COOKBOOK

A Beginner's Guide Recipes To Boost Fertility With Mediterranean Inspired Recipes And Pictures Included

CYNTHIA DORCAS

Copyright © [2024] by Cynthia Dorcas

All rights reserved. No part of this publication may be reproduced, distributed, or transmitted in any form or by any means, including photocopying, recording, or other electronic or mechanical methods, without the prior written permission of the publisher, except in the case of brief quotations embodied in critical reviews and certain other noncommercial uses permitted by copyright law.

TABLE OF CONTENT

CHAPTER 1 11
    What is IVF? 11
    The Role of Nutrition in IVF Success 11
    Importance of a Balanced Diet Before and During IVF 12
    Foods to Include in an IVF Diet 13
    Foods to Avoid in an IVF Diet 14

CHAPTER 2 16
BREAKFAST RECIPE 16
    Fertility-Boosting Avocado and Egg Toast .. 16
    Chia Seed and Almond Butter Smoothie Bowl 17
    Sweet Potato Breakfast Hash with Eggs 18
    Berry and Oat Breakfast Parfait 19
    Quinoa Breakfast Bowl with Almonds and Apples 20
    Spinach and Feta Omelet 20
    Overnight Oats with Flaxseeds and Berries 21
    Banana and Walnut Pancakes 22
    Pumpkin Seed and Yogurt Parfait 23
    Protein-Packed Tofu Scramble 24

CHAPTER 3 25
LUNCH RECIPES 25
    Quinoa and Avocado Salad with Lemon Tahini Dressing 25
    Lentil and Spinach Soup 26
    Grilled Chicken and Kale Salad with Pumpkin Seeds 27
    Roasted Vegetable and Farro Bowl 27
    Chickpea and Avocado Wrap 28
    Salmon and Quinoa Salad with Lemon Vinaigrette 29
    Tofu Stir-Fry with Broccoli and Cashews ... 30
    Beet and Goat Cheese Salad with Walnuts 31
    Black Bean and Sweet Potato Bowl 32
    Grilled Shrimp Salad with Avocado and Lime 33

CHAPTER 4 34
DINNERS RECIPES 34
    Baked Salmon with Asparagus and Quinoa 34
    Turkey and Zucchini Meatballs with Tomato Sauce 35
    Lentil and Sweet Potato Curry 36
    Grilled Chicken with Roasted Vegetables .. 37
    Cod with Spinach and White Beans 38
    Eggplant and Chickpea Stew 39
    Shrimp Stir-Fry with Broccoli and Cashews 40

Chicken and Sweet Potato Bake 41

Quinoa-Stuffed Bell Peppers 41

Grilled Tofu with Roasted Brussels Sprouts 42

CHAPTER 5 43

SNACKS AND DESSERTS RECIPES 43

Almond and Chia Seed Energy Bites 43

Greek Yogurt with Pumpkin Seeds and Berries 44

Roasted Chickpeas with Spices 45

Apple Slices with Almond Butter 46

Hard-Boiled Eggs with Avocado 46

Trail Mix with Walnuts, Dark Chocolate, and Dried Fruit 47

Celery Sticks with Hummus 48

Cottage Cheese with Pineapple 49

Carrot and Cucumber Sticks with Tahini Dip 49

Banana and Peanut Butter Smoothie 50

Dark Chocolate Avocado Mousse 51

Baked Apples with Cinnamon and Walnuts 52

Chia Pudding with Coconut and Mango ... 52

Almond Flour Brownies 53

Berry Crumble with Oats and Almonds 54

Coconut Macaroons 55

Chocolate-Covered Strawberries 56

Lemon and Blueberry Greek Yogurt Popsicles 57

No-Bake Peanut Butter Bars 58

Banana Nice Cream 58

CHAPTER 6 59

SOUP AND STEW RECIPES 59

Lentil and Vegetable Soup 59

Chicken and Sweet Potato Stew 60

Butternut Squash and Ginger Soup 61

Black Bean and Corn Chili 62

Carrot and Red Lentil Soup 63

Spinach and White Bean Soup 64

Thai Coconut Chicken Soup 65

Tomato and Basil Soup 65

Moroccan Chickpea Stew 66

Kale and Quinoa Soup 67

CHAPTER 7 69

4-Week Meal Plan for IVF Mothers 69

Week 1 69

Day 1 69

Breakfast: 69

Lunch: 69

Dinner: 69

Snack: 69	Dinner: 70
Day 2 69	Snack: 70
Breakfast: 69	Day 7 70
Lunch: 69	Breakfast: 70
Dinner: 69	Lunch: 70
Snack: 69	Dinner: 70
Day 3 69	Snack: 70
Breakfast: 69	Week 2 70
Lunch: 69	Day 1 70
Dinner: 69	Breakfast: 70
Snack: 69	Lunch: 70
Day 4 69	Dinner: 70
Breakfast: 69	Snack: 70
Lunch: 69	Day 2 70
Dinner: 69	Breakfast: 70
Snack: 69	Lunch: 70
Day 5 70	Dinner: 70
Breakfast: 70	Snack: 71
Lunch: 70	Day 3 71
Dinner: 70	Breakfast: 71
Snack: 70	Lunch: 71
Day 6 70	Dinner: 71
Breakfast: 70	Snack: 71
Lunch: 70	Day 4 71

Breakfast: 71
Lunch: 71
Dinner: 71
Snack: 71
    Day 5 71
Breakfast: 71
Lunch: 71
Dinner: 71
Snack: 71
    Day 6 71
Breakfast: 71
Lunch: 71
Dinner: 71
Snack: 71
    Day 7 71
Breakfast: 71
Lunch: 71
Dinner: 71
Snack: 72
    Week 3 72
    Day 1 72
Breakfast: 72
Lunch: 72
Dinner: 72

Snack: 72
    Day 2 72
Breakfast: 72
Lunch: 72
Dinner: 72
Snack: 72
    Day 3 72
Breakfast: 72
Lunch: 72
Dinner: 72
Snack: 72
    Day 4 72
Breakfast: 72
Lunch: 72
Dinner: 72
Snack: 72
    Day 5 72
Breakfast: 72
Lunch: 72
Dinner: 73
Snack: 73
    Day 6 73
Breakfast: 73
Lunch: 73

Dinner: 73
    Day 7 73
Breakfast: 73
Lunch: 73
Dinner: 73
Snack: 73
    Week 4 73
    Day 1 73
Breakfast: 73
Lunch: 73
Dinner: 73
Snack: 73
    Day 2 73
Breakfast: 73
Lunch: 73
Dinner: 73
Snack: 73
    Day 3 73
Breakfast: 73
Lunch: 74
Dinner: 74
Snack: 74
    Day 4 74
Breakfast: 74

Lunch: 74
Dinner: 74
Snack: 74
    Day 5 74
Breakfast: 74
Lunch: 74
Dinner: 74
Snack: 74
    Day 6 74
Breakfast: 74
Lunch: 74
Dinner: 74
Snack: 74
    Day 7 74
Breakfast: 74
Lunch: 74
Dinner: 74
Snack: 74
SHOPPING LIST 75
    Fruits: 75
    Vegetables: 75
    Grains: 75
    Proteins: 75
    Dairy or Dairy Alternatives: 75

Nuts & Seeds: 76

Condiments & Oils: 76

Spices & Seasonings: 76

Special Ingredients: 76

INTRODUCTION

Welcome to the **IVF Diet Cookbook**, a heartfelt guide to nourishing your body and mind as you embark on one of life's most important journeys—In Vitro Fertilization (IVF). Whether you are just beginning to explore fertility treatments or are in the middle of the IVF process, this book is designed to be your companion, offering practical advice, delicious recipes, and nutritional guidance to support you every step of the way.

Going through IVF can be both exciting and overwhelming. It's a time filled with hope, but it also brings with it unique challenges that can feel physically, emotionally, and mentally demanding. One thing that remains constant throughout this journey, however, is the power of the food you eat. What you choose to put into your body can make a real difference, not only in how you feel day-to-day but also in how your body responds to IVF treatment. Nutrition plays a critical role in supporting your reproductive health, improving egg quality, balancing hormones, and creating an environment that can enhance the chances of a successful pregnancy.

This book is not just about what to eat; it's about how to nourish yourself holistically during a time when your body needs it most. You'll find recipes that are tailored to the specific needs of women undergoing IVF, with a focus on whole, nutrient-dense ingredients that promote fertility and support your overall well-being. Whether it's a soothing smoothie packed with antioxidants to start your day or a hearty, nutrient-rich dinner that comforts your soul, the recipes in this book are designed to be simple, delicious, and filled with the nutrients you need.

But we're not just talking about physical nourishment. The IVF Diet Cookbook is also about caring for yourself emotionally. IVF can be a rollercoaster of emotions, and stress can sometimes feel like a constant companion. That's why we've included tips on mindful eating, managing stress through food, and finding comfort in meals that bring you joy.

Throughout these pages, you'll discover the vital role nutrition plays in every stage of IVF—before, during, and after embryo transfer. We'll explore the foods that can boost fertility, the nutrients your body needs during the different phases of treatment, and what to avoid to give yourself the best chance of success. You'll also find practical meal plans, easy-to-follow tips, and evidence-based advice to guide you as you nourish your body in preparation for this life-changing journey.

At the heart of this book is a message of empowerment. IVF is a process that can sometimes feel out of your control, but the one thing you can control is how you treat and nourish your body. With the right nutrition, you're giving yourself the best possible foundation to support your fertility, your health, and your future.

So, whether you're planning your meals in preparation for an IVF cycle or looking for ways to support your body post-transfer, this cookbook will serve as a trusted resource to help you feel empowered, supported, and nourished—every step of the way. Let's start this journey together, one meal at a time.

CHAPTER 1

What is IVF?

In Vitro Fertilization, commonly known as IVF, is a medical procedure used to help individuals or couples who are facing challenges with conception. Think of it as a process where science gives nature a little nudge. In simple terms, IVF involves retrieving mature eggs from a woman's ovaries and fertilizing them with sperm in a lab. Once fertilized, the egg (now an embryo) is transferred back into the woman's uterus with the hope that it will implant and grow into a healthy pregnancy.

For many people, IVF is a journey full of hope, patience, and care. It can be a lifeline for those who have struggled to conceive naturally. While the process is complex and can sometimes feel overwhelming, it's also a time when nutrition and lifestyle choices become crucial to boosting the chances of success.

During the IVF process, your body is doing a lot of work. Medications are used to stimulate the ovaries to produce more eggs than usual, and your body is preparing for the possibility of pregnancy. This means your body needs the right kind of fuel to help everything run smoothly. And that's where diet comes in. You might be surprised at just how much what you eat can influence the outcome of your IVF cycle.

The Role of Nutrition in IVF Success

We often hear the saying, "you are what you eat," and when it comes to IVF, this couldn't be truer. Nutrition plays a significant role in supporting the body during IVF, not only in preparing for the procedure but also in helping with egg quality, hormonal balance, and even the likelihood of a successful pregnancy.

Let's break it down a little. When you're going through IVF, your body is trying to produce multiple eggs at once, which is not something it does during a typical monthly cycle. To make sure your eggs are healthy and ready for fertilization, your body needs plenty of nutrients, antioxidants, and vitamins to protect the cells and keep things functioning optimally.

For instance, folate (the natural form of folic acid) is incredibly important for women trying to conceive. It helps prevent neural tube defects in the developing baby, but it's also essential for healthy cell division during egg formation. That's why many fertility experts recommend increasing your intake of leafy greens like spinach and kale, which are high in folate.

Then there are omega-3 fatty acids, often found in fatty fish like salmon or in plant-based sources like chia seeds and walnuts. These healthy fats are anti-inflammatory and help regulate hormone production, which is key to creating a healthy environment for conception.

The IVF process can be stressful, both physically and emotionally, and stress can affect your body's ability to respond well to treatment. Eating foods rich in magnesium, such as almonds, seeds, and avocados, can help regulate your stress levels and improve your mood. This is important because stress hormones like cortisol can interfere with reproductive hormones like progesterone, which is crucial for maintaining a pregnancy.

Don't forget about hydration. Drinking plenty of water keeps your body's systems running smoothly, including hormone transport and egg health. Dehydration can affect your cervical fluid, making it less hospitable to sperm and embryos. So, while it's easy to focus solely on what you're eating, don't underestimate the power of simply staying hydrated.

Importance of a Balanced Diet Before and During IVF

So, what exactly does a balanced diet look like before and during IVF? Well, think of it as creating the perfect environment for a little seed to grow. You need good soil (your body) and the right nutrients to ensure that everything is in place for that seed to sprout and flourish.

First, let's talk about protein. Protein is essential for the production of hormones like oestrogen and progesterone, which are key players in your reproductive system. Good sources of protein include lean meats, poultry, fish, eggs, and plant-based options like lentils, beans, and quinoa. It's a good idea to make sure you're getting a healthy balance of both animal and plant-based proteins to support your body.

Complex carbohydrates, like whole grains, sweet potatoes, and brown rice, provide a slow and steady release of energy, which is important when your body is working hard. Unlike refined carbohydrates (think white bread and sugary snacks), complex carbs won't cause your blood sugar to spike and crash. This is important because unstable blood sugar can mess with your hormone levels, which can affect your IVF treatment.

Healthy fats, as we mentioned earlier, are also essential. These include foods like avocados, olive oil, nuts, and seeds. Healthy fats help to keep inflammation in check, support hormone production, and improve the absorption of fat-soluble vitamins like A, D, E, and K. All of these are essential for maintaining a healthy reproductive system.

Vegetables, especially the dark green and brightly coloured ones, are packed with antioxidants, vitamins, and minerals that protect your cells from oxidative stress. During IVF, your body is producing eggs, and you want to make sure that the environment in which they're developing is as healthy as possible. Antioxidants help fight off free radicals, which can damage cells and reduce egg quality.

Fibre is another key component of a balanced diet. Fibre-rich foods like whole grains, fruits, and vegetables help regulate digestion and remove excess hormones, such as oestrogen, from the body. This is particularly important because too much or too little oestrogen can interfere with your IVF treatment and overall hormonal balance.

It's also important to reduce the intake of processed and sugary foods. These can lead to inflammation in the body and disrupt your blood sugar levels, which in turn can affect your hormonal balance. Instead, opt for whole, unprocessed foods that nourish your body and support your reproductive health.

And of course, let's not forget about hydration. Drinking enough water is often overlooked but is critical for supporting all bodily functions, including reproduction. Water helps to flush toxins from the body, keep your cells hydrated, and ensure that your blood (which carries nutrients) is flowing efficiently.

Lastly, consider incorporating some fertility-boosting foods into your diet. For example, Brazil nuts are a great source of selenium, a mineral that helps to improve sperm motility and support egg quality. Dark chocolate (in moderation!) is high in antioxidants and can even improve blood flow, which is important for a healthy uterus

Foods to Include in an IVF Diet

When going through IVF, it's important to nourish your body with foods that support fertility, egg quality, and overall well-being. Here are five key foods that are beneficial for your IVF journey:

Leafy Greens (Spinach, Kale, Swiss Chard)

Leafy greens are packed with essential nutrients, particularly folate, which is vital for both men and women during fertility treatments. Folate aids in cell division and DNA replication, which is especially important during egg and embryo development. These vegetables are also high in fibre, iron, and antioxidants, which help reduce inflammation and protect cells from oxidative damage.

Fatty Fish (Salmon, Mackerel, Sardines)

Fatty fish like salmon, mackerel, and sardines are rich in omega-3 fatty acids, which are known to promote reproductive health. Omega-3s help reduce inflammation, regulate hormone production, and improve blood flow to reproductive organs. These healthy fats also support embryo implantation and overall pregnancy health.

Eggs

Eggs are an excellent source of high-quality protein and essential nutrients like choline, which is important for brain development in early pregnancy. They also provide healthy fats and vitamins that support egg quality and hormone production, which are crucial during the IVF process.

Nuts and Seeds (Walnuts, Chia Seeds, Flaxseeds)

Nuts and seeds are packed with nutrients that support fertility, such as healthy fats, protein, and antioxidants. Walnuts, for example, are particularly high in omega-3 fatty acids, while chia and flaxseeds provide fibre and lignans, which help balance hormones and improve reproductive health.

Berries (Blueberries, Raspberries, Strawberries)

Berries are rich in antioxidants, which protect your cells from oxidative stress and improve overall reproductive health. They are also high in fibre, which helps balance hormones by eliminating excess oestrogen from the body. Berries provide a natural source of sweetness without spiking blood sugar levels, making them a perfect fertility-friendly food.

Foods to Avoid in an IVF Diet

While there are many foods that support fertility, there are also some that can hinder your IVF journey. Here are five foods to limit or avoid during your treatment:

Processed Foods

Processed foods, such as packaged snacks, fast food, and ready-made meals, often contain unhealthy trans fats, high levels of sodium, and added sugars. These ingredients can lead to inflammation, disrupt hormonal balance, and negatively affect egg and sperm quality. They also tend to lack essential nutrients that your body needs during IVF.

Refined Sugars

Refined sugars, found in sweets, sodas, and many baked goods, can cause blood sugar spikes and crashes, which disrupt hormone levels. A diet high in refined sugars can also increase the risk of developing insulin resistance, which can interfere with ovulation and overall fertility. Excess sugar consumption can also contribute to weight gain, another factor that may negatively impact IVF outcomes.

Excessive Caffeine

While a small amount of caffeine (around 200 mg per day) is generally considered safe, excessive caffeine intake can be harmful to fertility. Too much caffeine can interfere with hormone levels, increase the risk of miscarriage, and reduce the chances of a successful implantation after embryo transfer.

Alcohol

Alcohol is best avoided entirely during the IVF process. Even moderate drinking can affect fertility by disrupting hormone levels, reducing sperm quality, and increasing the risk of miscarriage. For women undergoing IVF, alcohol can also impair egg quality and interfere with the success of the treatment.

High-Mercury Fish (Tuna, Swordfish, King Mackerel)

While fish is generally a great source of omega-3s and protein, certain types of fish that are high in mercury should be avoided during IVF. Mercury can build up in the body and affect reproductive health, potentially harming egg quality and increasing the risk of developmental issues in early pregnancy.

CHAPTER 2

BREAKFAST RECIPE

Fertility-Boosting Avocado and Egg Toast

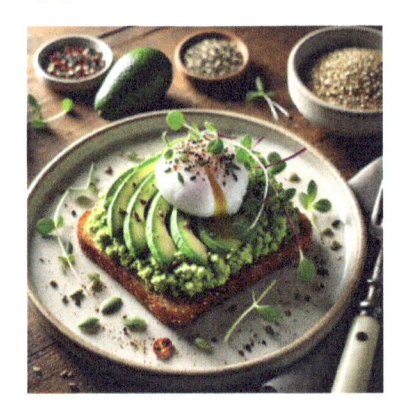

Servings: 1

Cooking Time: 10 minutes

Ingredients:

- 1 slice whole-grain or sprouted bread
- 1/2 ripe avocado, mashed
- 1 large egg (organic, if possible)
- 1 teaspoon olive oil
- Salt and pepper to taste
- Red pepper flakes or fresh herbs for garnish (optional)

Instructions:

- Toast the slice of bread to your desired crispiness.
- While the bread is toasting, heat the olive oil in a small pan over medium heat. Crack the egg into the pan and cook until the whites are set, but the yolk is still runny (or to your preference).
- Spread the mashed avocado onto the toast and top with the cooked egg.
- Season with salt, pepper, and a pinch of red pepper flakes or fresh herbs.
- Serve immediately for a quick, nutrient-rich breakfast that supports fertility.

Nutritional Information (per serving):

- Calories: 280 kcal
- Protein: 10g
- Fat: 21g
- Carbohydrates: 16g
- Fiber: 7g
- Vitamin A: 8% RDA
- Folate: 30% RDA
- Omega-3: 200 mg

Nutritional Benefits:

Eggs are rich in choline and vitamin D, both of which play a vital role in supporting fertility and egg quality. Avocados provide healthy monounsaturated fats that help regulate hormone levels, making this a perfect fertility-boosting breakfast.

Chia Seed and Almond Butter Smoothie Bowl

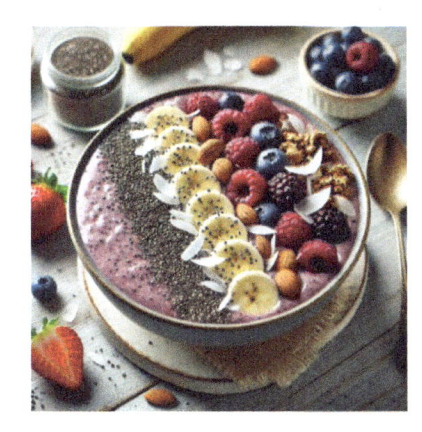

Servings: 1

Cooking Time: 10 minutes (plus 4 hours chilling time for chia pudding)

Ingredients:

- 1/4 cup chia seeds
- 1 cup unsweetened almond milk
- 1 tablespoon almond butter
- 1/2 banana
- 1 teaspoon honey or maple syrup (optional)
- 1/4 cup granola
- Fresh berries and coconut flakes for topping

Instructions:

- In a jar or bowl, combine the chia seeds and almond milk. Stir well and refrigerate for at least 4 hours, or overnight, to allow the chia seeds to thicken.
- Once the chia pudding is ready, blend the chia mixture with the almond butter, banana, and honey until smooth and creamy.
- Pour the smoothie mixture into a bowl and top with granola, fresh berries, and coconut flakes.
- Enjoy a filling and nourishing smoothie bowl that will keep you energized and satisfied.

Nutritional Information (per serving):

- Calories: 450 kcal
- Protein: 12g
- Fat: 28g
- Carbohydrates: 40g
- Fiber: 14g
- Omega-3: 5g
- Calcium: 300 mg
- Vitamin C: 15% RDA

Nutritional Benefits:

Chia seeds are loaded with omega-3 fatty acids and fiber, making them an excellent addition to a fertility-friendly diet. Almond butter provides a source of protein and vitamin E, which is known to improve egg quality.

Sweet Potato Breakfast Hash with Eggs

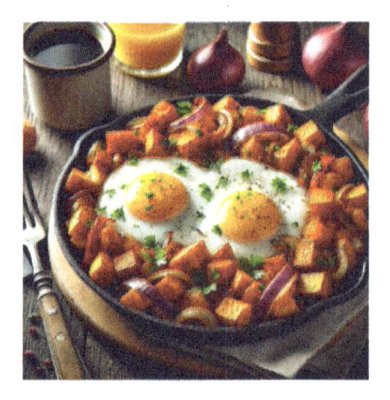

Servings: 1

Cooking Time: 25 minutes

Ingredients:

- 1 medium sweet potato, peeled and diced
- 1/4 red bell pepper, diced
- 1/4 onion, diced
- 2 large eggs
- 1 tablespoon olive oil
- Salt and pepper to taste
- Fresh parsley for garnish

Instructions:

- Heat the olive oil in a large skillet over medium heat. Add the diced sweet potatoes and cook for 10 minutes, stirring occasionally, until they start to soften.
- Add the bell pepper and onion to the skillet, and cook for an additional 5-7 minutes until all vegetables are tender and lightly browned.
- In a separate pan, fry or scramble the eggs to your liking.
- Season the sweet potato hash with salt and pepper, and serve it with the eggs on top. Garnish with fresh parsley, if desired.
- This hearty breakfast will provide sustained energy and support fertility with its rich nutrient content.

Nutritional Information (per serving):

- Calories: 350 kcal
- Protein: 10g
- Fat: 20g
- Carbohydrates: 30g
- Fiber: 7g
- Vitamin A: 200% RDA
- Folate: 25% RDA
- Iron: 10% RDA

Nutritional Benefits:

Sweet potatoes are a rich source of beta-carotene and vitamin A, which can help support healthy progesterone levels. This breakfast hash provides protein from eggs and healthy fats from olive oil, making it an excellent choice for fertility.

Berry and Oat Breakfast Parfait

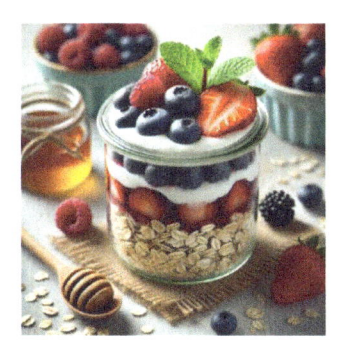

Servings: 1

Cooking Time: 10 minutes

Ingredients:

- 1/2 cup rolled oats
- 1/2 cup plain Greek yogurt (or a dairy-free alternative)
- 1 tablespoon chia seeds
- 1/2 cup mixed fresh berries (blueberries, raspberries, strawberries)
- 1 teaspoon honey or maple syrup (optional)

Instructions:

- In a small bowl or jar, layer the rolled oats, Greek yogurt, and chia seeds.
- Top with fresh berries and drizzle with honey or maple syrup if desired.
- Let the parfait sit for a few minutes to allow the chia seeds to thicken slightly, or prepare the night before and refrigerate for a grab-and-go breakfast.
- Enjoy this fiber-rich and antioxidant-packed parfait that supports fertility and digestion.

Nutritional Information (per serving):

- Calories: 250 kcal
- Protein: 10g
- Fat: 6g
- Carbohydrates: 42g
- Fiber: 8g
- Calcium: 15% RDA
- Antioxidants: High from berries

Nutritional Benefits:

Oats are a great source of fiber and slow-digesting carbohydrates that help maintain steady blood sugar levels, which is important for hormonal balance. Berries are packed with antioxidants, making them a fertility-boosting powerhouse.

Quinoa Breakfast Bowl with Almonds and Apples

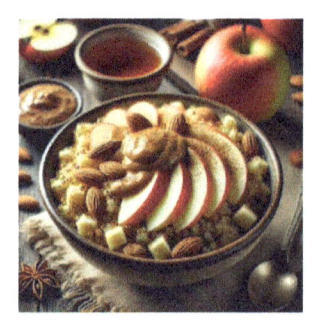

Servings: 1

Cooking Time: 10 minutes (plus cooking quinoa)

Ingredients:

- 1/2 cup cooked quinoa
- 1/2 apple, diced
- 1 tablespoon almond butter
- 1 tablespoon slivered almonds
- 1 teaspoon cinnamon
- 1 teaspoon honey or maple syrup (optional)

Instructions:

- In a small saucepan, warm the cooked quinoa over low heat.
- Once the quinoa is heated, stir in the almond butter and cinnamon until well combined.
- Transfer the quinoa to a bowl and top with diced apple, slivered almonds, and a drizzle of honey or maple syrup.
- Serve warm for a cozy and nourishing breakfast that supports fertility with its nutrient-dense ingredients.

Nutritional Information (per serving):

- Calories: 330 kcal
- Protein: 10g
- Fat: 16g
- Carbohydrates: 40g
- Fiber: 8g
- Iron: 15% RDA
- Vitamin E: 20% RDA

Nutritional Benefits:

Quinoa is a complete protein and provides a rich source of magnesium and folate, both important for reproductive health. Almonds add vitamin E and healthy fats, while apples provide fiber and antioxidants.

Spinach and Feta Omelet

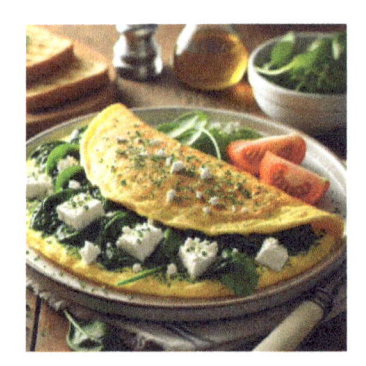

Servings: 1

Cooking Time: 10 minutes

Ingredients:

- 2 large eggs
- 1/4 cup fresh spinach, chopped
- 2 tablespoons crumbled feta cheese
- 1 tablespoon olive oil
- Salt and pepper to taste

Instructions:

- Heat the olive oil in a small non-stick pan over medium heat.
- In a small bowl, whisk the eggs with a pinch of salt and pepper.
- Pour the egg mixture into the pan and cook for 1-2 minutes until the eggs begin to set.
- Sprinkle the chopped spinach and feta cheese over one half of the omelet.
- Fold the other half of the omelet over the filling and cook for another minute until the eggs are fully cooked.
- Serve immediately for a protein-rich and fertility-friendly breakfast.

Nutritional Information (per serving):

- Calories: 250 kcal
- Protein: 16g
- Fat: 20g
- Carbohydrates: 3g
- Fiber: 1g
- Folate: 35% RDA
- Calcium: 15% RDA

Nutritional Benefits:

Spinach is loaded with folate, which is crucial for egg development and early pregnancy. Feta cheese provides calcium and protein, making this omelet a balanced and nutrient-dense start to the day.

Overnight Oats with Flaxseeds and Berries

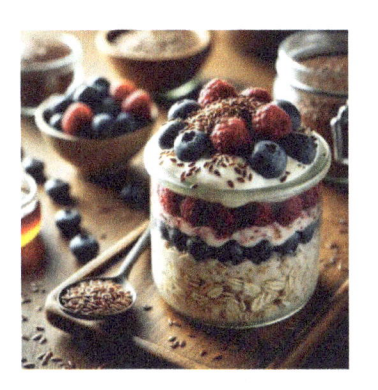

Servings: 1

Cooking Time: 5 minutes (plus overnight soaking)

Ingredients:

- 1/2 cup rolled oats
- 1 tablespoon flaxseeds
- 1/2 cup unsweetened almond milk
- 1/2 teaspoon vanilla extract
- 1/2 cup mixed fresh or frozen berries
- 1 teaspoon honey or maple syrup (optional)

Instructions:

- In a jar or bowl, combine the oats, flaxseeds, almond milk, and vanilla extract. Stir well to combine.
- Cover and refrigerate overnight.
- In the morning, top the oats with berries and drizzle with honey or maple syrup if desired.
- Enjoy this easy, make-ahead breakfast that's rich in fertility-supporting ingredients.

Nutritional Information (per serving):

- Calories: 280 kcal
- Protein: 8g
- Fat: 10g
- Carbohydrates: 40g
- Fiber: 10g
- Omega-3: 2g
- Calcium: 15% RDA

Nutritional Benefits:

Flaxseeds are a rich source of omega-3 fatty acids and fiber, both of which are essential for hormone balance and fertility. The oats and berries add fiber and antioxidants, making this a complete breakfast.

Banana and Walnut Pancakes

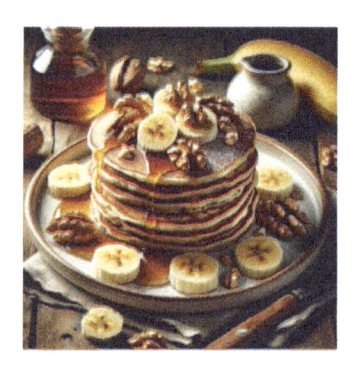

Servings: 1

Cooking Time: 15 minutes

Ingredients:

- 1 ripe banana, mashed
- 1 large egg
- 1/4 cup rolled oats
- 1/4 teaspoon cinnamon
- 1 tablespoon chopped walnuts
- 1 tablespoon olive oil for cooking

Instructions:

- In a bowl, mash the banana and mix it with the egg, oats, and cinnamon until well combined.
- Heat the olive oil in a non-stick skillet over medium heat.
- Pour small amounts of the batter into the skillet to form pancakes and cook for 2-3 minutes on each side until golden brown.

- Serve with a sprinkle of chopped walnuts and a drizzle of honey for a nutrient-packed breakfast.

Nutritional Information (per serving):

- Calories: 300 kcal
- Protein: 8g
- Fat: 14g
- Carbohydrates: 38g
- Fiber: 6g
- Potassium: 15% RDA
- Omega-3: 150 mg

Nutritional Benefits:

Bananas are rich in potassium and vitamin B6, which help regulate hormones, while walnuts provide a healthy dose of omega-3 fatty acids and antioxidants, both essential for reproductive health.

Pumpkin Seed and Yogurt Parfait

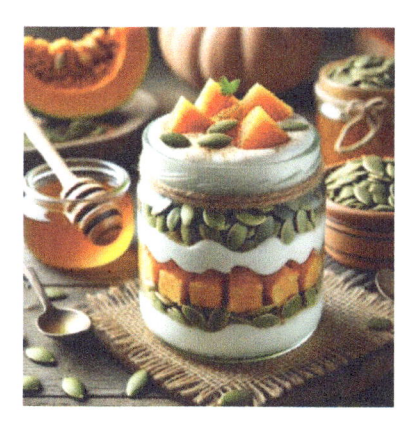

Servings: 1

Cooking Time: 5 minutes

Ingredients:

- 1/2 cup plain Greek yogurt (or dairy-free alternative)
- 2 tablespoons pumpkin seeds
- 1 tablespoon chia seeds
- 1/4 cup fresh or dried cranberries
- 1 teaspoon honey or maple syrup (optional)

Instructions:

- In a bowl or jar, layer the yogurt with pumpkin seeds, chia seeds, and cranberries.
- Drizzle with honey or maple syrup if desired.
- Enjoy this quick and easy parfait that supports both gut health and fertility.

Nutritional Information (per serving):

- Calories: 230 kcal
- Protein: 12g
- Fat: 12g
- Carbohydrates: 20g
- Fiber: 5g
- Zinc: 20% RDA
- Calcium: 15% RDA

Nutritional Benefits:

Pumpkin seeds are an excellent source of zinc, which supports fertility by improving sperm quality and ovulation. The yogurt provides probiotics, which are important for gut health and hormone regulation.

Protein-Packed Tofu Scramble

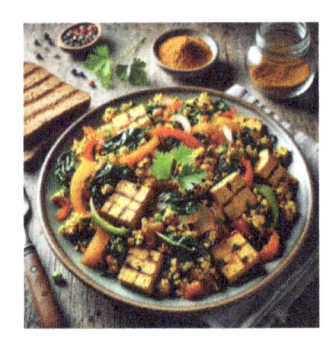

Servings: 1

Cooking Time: 10 minutes

Ingredients:

- 1/2 block firm tofu, crumbled
- 1/4 red bell pepper, diced
- 1/4 cup spinach, chopped
- 1/4 onion, diced
- 1 tablespoon olive oil
- 1/2 teaspoon turmeric
- Salt and pepper to taste

Instructions:

- Heat the olive oil in a pan over medium heat. Add the onion and bell pepper, and sauté until softened.
- Add the crumbled tofu, spinach, turmeric, salt, and pepper. Cook for 5-7 minutes, stirring occasionally, until the tofu is heated through and the spinach is wilted.
- Serve hot for a plant-based, protein-rich breakfast that supports hormonal balance and fertility.

Nutritional Information (per serving):

- Calories: 200 kcal
- Protein: 12g
- Fat: 14g
- Carbohydrates: 10g
- Fiber: 3g
- Iron: 20% RDA
- Calcium: 15% RDA

Nutritional Benefits:

Tofu is a great plant-based protein source and contains phytoestrogens that help balance hormones. Paired with vegetables, this scramble provides a nutrient-dense, fertility-friendly breakfast.

CHAPTER 3

LUNCH RECIPES

Quinoa and Avocado Salad with Lemon Tahini Dressing

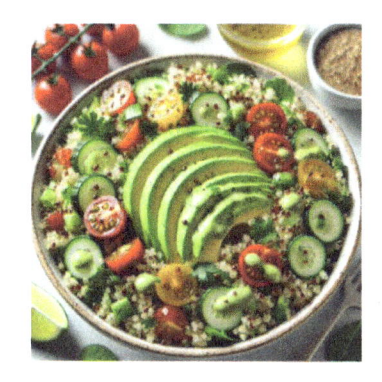

Servings: 1

Cooking Time: 20 minutes

Ingredients:

- 1 cup cooked quinoa
- 1/2 ripe avocado, sliced
- 1/2 cup cherry tomatoes, halved
- 1/4 cup cucumber, diced
- 2 tablespoons fresh parsley, chopped
- 2 tablespoons tahini
- 1 tablespoon lemon juice
- 1 tablespoon olive oil
- Salt and pepper to taste

Instructions:

- In a large bowl, combine the cooked quinoa, avocado, cherry tomatoes, cucumber, and parsley.
- In a small bowl, whisk together the tahini, lemon juice, olive oil, salt, and pepper to make the dressing.
- Drizzle the dressing over the salad and toss gently to combine.
- Serve immediately for a fresh, nutrient-dense lunch that supports fertility and energy levels.

Nutritional Information (per serving):

- Calories: 350 kcal
- Protein: 8g
- Fat: 25g
- Carbohydrates: 28g
- Fiber: 8g
- Folate: 25% RDA
- Iron: 12% RDA

Nutritional Benefits:

Quinoa is a complete protein that provides all nine essential amino acids, making it ideal for maintaining energy levels and supporting tissue growth. Avocado adds healthy fats, which are important for hormonal health, and the lemon-tahini dressing offers a burst of antioxidants and calcium.

Lentil and Spinach Soup

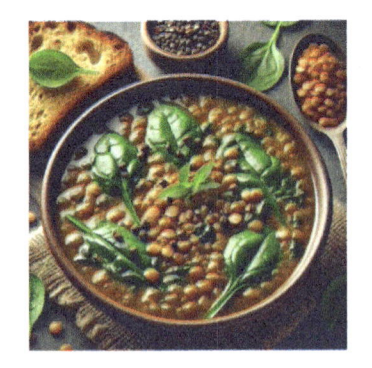

Servings: 1

Cooking Time: 30 minutes

Ingredients:

- 1 cup dried lentils, rinsed
- 4 cups vegetable broth
- 1 cup fresh spinach, chopped
- 1 onion, diced
- 2 garlic cloves, minced
- 1 tablespoon olive oil
- 1 teaspoon cumin
- 1/2 teaspoon turmeric
- Salt and pepper to taste

Instructions:

- Heat the olive oil in a large pot over medium heat. Add the onion and garlic, and sauté until softened.
- Add the lentils, cumin, turmeric, and vegetable broth to the pot. Bring to a boil, then reduce the heat and simmer for 20-25 minutes until the lentils are tender.
- Stir in the chopped spinach and cook for an additional 5 minutes.
- Season with salt and pepper, and serve warm. This comforting soup is perfect for supporting fertility with its rich nutrient content.

Nutritional Information (per serving):

- Calories: 200 kcal
- Protein: 10g
- Fat: 6g
- Carbohydrates: 32g
- Fiber: 14g
- Iron: 20% RDA
- Folate: 50% RDA

Nutritional Benefits:

Lentils are an excellent source of plant-based protein, iron, and folate, all of which are essential for reproductive health and fertility. Spinach adds a rich source of folate and iron, making this soup a hearty and nourishing meal for IVF mothers.

Grilled Chicken and Kale Salad with Pumpkin Seeds

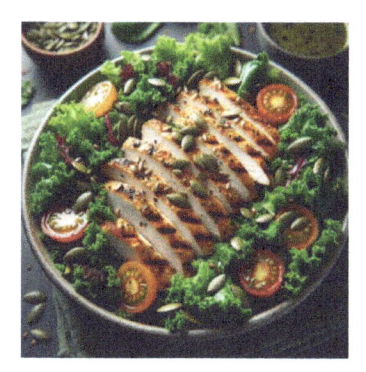

Servings: 1

Cooking Time: 15 minutes (excluding chicken grilling time)

Ingredients:

- 2 grilled chicken breasts, sliced
- 4 cups kale, chopped
- 1/4 cup pumpkin seeds
- 1/4 cup cherry tomatoes, halved
- 1 tablespoon olive oil
- 1 tablespoon lemon juice
- Salt and pepper to taste

Instructions:

- In a large bowl, massage the chopped kale with olive oil and lemon juice to soften the leaves.
- Add the grilled chicken, pumpkin seeds, and cherry tomatoes to the kale.
- Season with salt and pepper, and toss to combine.
- Serve immediately for a high-protein, nutrient-packed salad that supports fertility and overall health.

Nutritional Information (per serving):

- Calories: 350 kcal
- Protein: 30g
- Fat: 18g
- Carbohydrates: 12g
- Fiber: 5g
- Vitamin A: 120% RDA
- Calcium: 15% RDA

Nutritional Benefits:

Grilled chicken provides lean protein that supports muscle growth and tissue repair, both of which are important during IVF. Kale is rich in antioxidants, calcium, and folate, while pumpkin seeds add zinc and healthy fats that support hormone production.

Roasted Vegetable and Farro Bowl

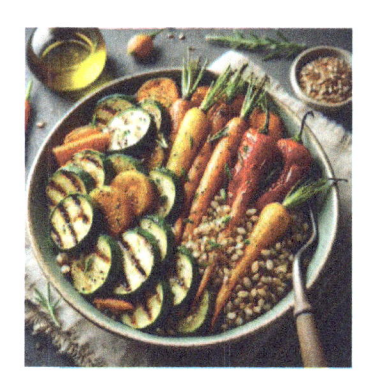

Servings: 1

Cooking Time: 40 minutes

Ingredients:

- 1 cup cooked farro
- 1 sweet potato, peeled and diced
- 1/2 red bell pepper, sliced
- 1/2 zucchini, sliced
- 2 tablespoons olive oil
- 1 teaspoon smoked paprika
- Salt and pepper to taste

Instructions:

- Preheat your oven to 400°F (200°C). Toss the sweet potato, bell pepper, and zucchini with olive oil, smoked paprika, salt, and pepper.
- Spread the vegetables on a baking sheet and roast for 25-30 minutes, stirring halfway through, until tender and caramelized.
- In a large bowl, combine the cooked farro and roasted vegetables. Toss to combine and serve warm for a hearty, nutrient-dense lunch that supports fertility and hormonal health.

Nutritional Information (per serving):

- Calories: 380 kcal
- Protein: 9g
- Fat: 16g
- Carbohydrates: 52g
- Fiber: 9g
- Vitamin A: 120% RDA
- Iron: 15% RDA

Nutritional Benefits:

Farro is an ancient grain that is high in fiber, protein, and iron, making it a fantastic choice for sustained energy and reproductive health. Roasted vegetables like sweet potatoes and bell peppers provide antioxidants and beta-carotene, which support egg quality and hormonal balance.

Chickpea and Avocado Wrap

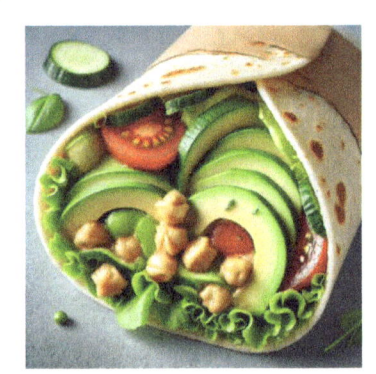

Servings: 1

Cooking Time: 10 minutes

Ingredients:

- 1 cup cooked chickpeas
- 1/2 ripe avocado, mashed
- 1/4 cup cucumber, sliced

- 1/4 cup shredded carrots
- 1 tablespoon tahini
- 1 teaspoon lemon juice
- 1 whole-grain tortilla
- Salt and pepper to taste

Instructions:

- In a small bowl, mash the chickpeas and avocado together. Stir in the tahini, lemon juice, salt, and pepper.
- Spread the chickpea mixture onto the whole-grain tortilla.
- Top with cucumber slices and shredded carrots.
- Roll the tortilla into a wrap and serve for a quick, protein-rich lunch that supports fertility.

Nutritional Information (per serving):

- Calories: 420 kcal
- Protein: 12g
- Fat: 22g
- Carbohydrates: 48g
- Fiber: 14g
- Folate: 35% RDA
- Iron: 20% RDA

Nutritional Benefits:

Chickpeas are a great source of plant-based protein, iron, and folate, all essential for reproductive health. Avocados provide healthy fats that support hormonal balance, while whole-grain tortillas offer fiber for digestion and energy.

Salmon and Quinoa Salad with Lemon Vinaigrette

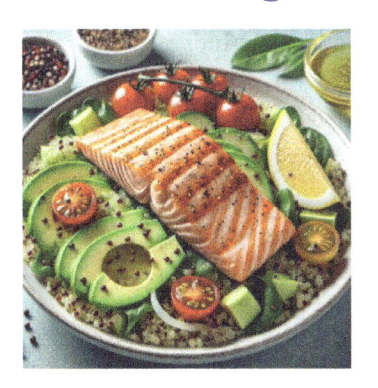

Servings: 1

Cooking Time: 20 minutes (excluding salmon grilling time)

Ingredients:

- 2 salmon fillets, grilled or baked
- 1 cup cooked quinoa
- 2 cups mixed greens
- 1/4 cup cucumber, sliced
- 2 tablespoons fresh parsley, chopped
- 1 tablespoon olive oil
- 1 tablespoon lemon juice
- Salt and pepper to taste

Instructions:

- In a large bowl, combine the cooked quinoa, mixed greens, cucumber, and parsley.
- Flake the cooked salmon and add it to the salad.
- In a small bowl, whisk together the olive oil, lemon juice, salt, and pepper to make the vinaigrette.
- Drizzle the vinaigrette over the salad and toss to combine. Serve immediately for a light, nutrient-packed lunch.

Nutritional Information (per serving):

- Calories: 450 kcal
- Protein: 32g
- Fat: 22g
- Carbohydrates: 28g
- Fiber: 6g
- Omega-3: 2g
- Vitamin C: 20% RDA

Nutritional Benefits:

Salmon is one of the best sources of omega-3 fatty acids, which reduce inflammation and support fertility. Quinoa provides a complete source of protein, while the lemon vinaigrette adds a burst of antioxidants and vitamin C.

Tofu Stir-Fry with Broccoli and Cashews

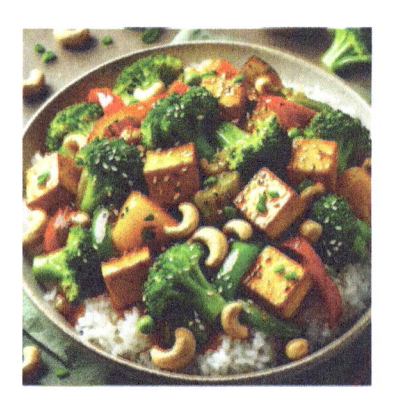

Servings: 1
Cooking Time: 20 minutes

Ingredients:

- 1 block firm tofu, cubed
- 1 cup broccoli florets
- 1/2 red bell pepper, sliced
- 1/4 cup cashews, chopped
- 2 tablespoons soy sauce (or tamari for gluten-free)
- 1 tablespoon sesame oil
- 1 garlic clove, minced
- 1 teaspoon grated fresh ginger

Instructions:

- Heat the sesame oil in a large skillet over medium heat. Add the garlic and ginger, and sauté until fragrant.
- Add the tofu, broccoli, and red bell pepper to the skillet, and stir-fry for 5-7 minutes

- until the vegetables are tender and the tofu is golden brown.
- Stir in the soy sauce and cashews, and cook for an additional 2 minutes.
- Serve hot for a satisfying, protein-rich lunch that supports fertility.

Nutritional Benefits:

Tofu is a great plant-based protein source that also contains phytoestrogens, which can help balance hormones. Broccoli is rich in antioxidants and fiber, while cashews provide zinc, which is important for reproductive health.

Beet and Goat Cheese Salad with Walnuts

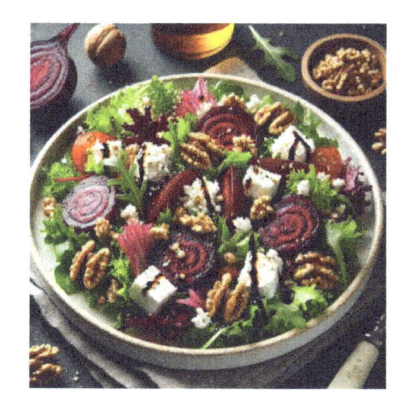

Servings: 1

Cooking Time: 55 minutes (including beet roasting time)

Ingredients:

- 2 medium beets, peeled and roasted
- 4 cups mixed greens (arugula, spinach, etc.)
- 1/4 cup crumbled goat cheese
- 1/4 cup walnuts, chopped
- 1 tablespoon balsamic vinegar
- 1 teaspoon honey
- Salt and pepper to taste

Instructions:

- Preheat your oven to 400°F (200°C). Wrap the beets in foil and roast for 45-50 minutes until tender. Once cool, slice the beets into wedges.
- In a large bowl, combine the mixed greens, roasted beets, goat cheese, and walnuts.
- In a small bowl, whisk together the balsamic vinegar, honey, salt, and pepper.
- Drizzle the dressing over the salad and toss gently to combine. Serve immediately for a fresh, nutrient-rich lunch that supports fertility.

Nutritional Information (per serving):

- Calories: 320 kcal
- Protein: 10g
- Fat: 20g
- Carbohydrates: 28g
- Fiber: 6g
- Vitamin C: 15% RDA
- Calcium: 20% RDA

Nutritional Benefits:

Beets are a fantastic source of iron and folate, both essential for reproductive health. Goat cheese provides calcium and protein, while walnuts add omega-3 fatty acids and antioxidants that support fertility.

Black Bean and Sweet Potato Bowl

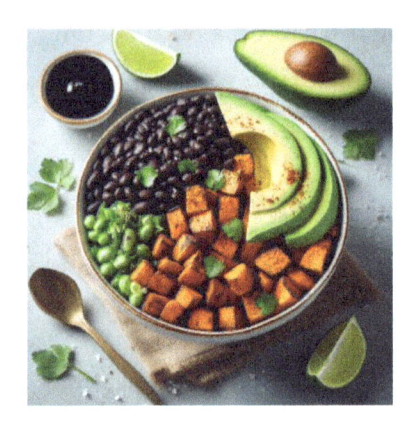

Servings: 1

Cooking Time: 30 minutes

Ingredients:

- 1 cup cooked black beans
- 1 sweet potato, peeled and diced
- 1/2 avocado, sliced
- 1/4 cup salsa
- 1 tablespoon olive oil
- 1 teaspoon cumin
- Salt and pepper to taste

Instructions:

- Preheat your oven to 400°F (200°C). Toss the diced sweet potatoes with olive oil, cumin, salt, and pepper. Roast for 25-30 minutes until tender.
- In a large bowl, combine the cooked black beans and roasted sweet potatoes.
- Top with avocado slices and salsa.
- Serve immediately for a filling, nutrient-dense lunch that supports fertility.

Nutritional Information (per serving):

- Calories: 400 kcal
- Protein: 12g
- Fat: 18g
- Carbohydrates: 55g
- Fiber: 16g
- Vitamin A: 100% RDA
- Folate: 25% RDA

Nutritional Benefits:

Black beans are rich in plant-based protein and fiber, while sweet potatoes provide beta-carotene, which is important for progesterone production. This bowl is packed with fertility-boosting nutrients and sustained energy.

Grilled Shrimp Salad with Avocado and Lime

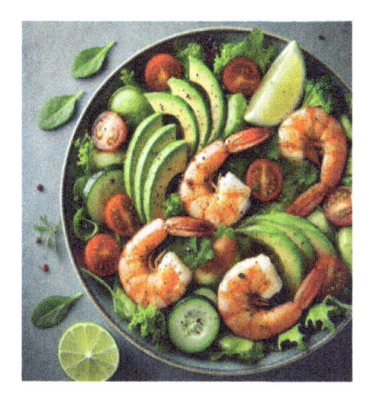

Servings: 1

Cooking Time: 15 minutes

Ingredients:

- 1/2-pound shrimp, peeled and deveined
- 2 cups mixed greens
- 1/2 avocado, sliced
- 1/4 cup cherry tomatoes, halved
- 1 tablespoon olive oil
- 1 tablespoon lime juice
- Salt and pepper to taste

Instructions:

- Heat the olive oil in a skillet over medium heat. Add the shrimp and cook for 2-3 minutes on each side until pink and cooked through.
- In a large bowl, combine the mixed greens, avocado, and cherry tomatoes.
- Add the cooked shrimp to the salad and drizzle with lime juice.
- Season with salt and pepper, toss gently, and serve immediately for a light, fertility-friendly lunch.

Nutritional Information (per serving):

- Calories: 300 kcal
- Protein: 24g
- Fat: 18g
- Carbohydrates: 10g
- Fiber: 5g
- Omega-3: 1g
- Vitamin C: 25% RDA

Nutritional Benefits:

Shrimp is a lean source of protein and provides selenium, a mineral that plays a key role in reproductive health. Avocado adds healthy fats, while the lime dressing provides antioxidants and vitamin C.

CHAPTER 4

DINNERS RECIPES

Baked Salmon with Asparagus and Quinoa

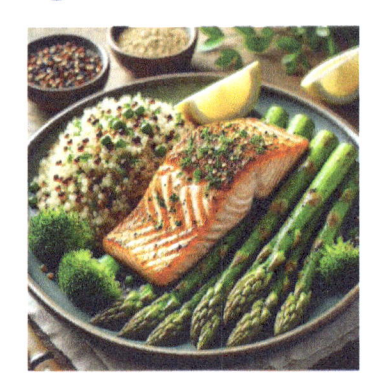

Servings: 1

Cooking Time: 25 minutes

Ingredients:

- 2 salmon fillets
- 1 bunch asparagus, trimmed
- 1 cup cooked quinoa
- 2 tablespoons olive oil
- 1 lemon, sliced
- 1 garlic clove, minced
- Salt and pepper to taste

Instructions:

- Preheat the oven to 375°F (190°C). Place the salmon fillets and asparagus on a baking sheet.
- Drizzle with olive oil, sprinkle with minced garlic, and season with salt and pepper.
- Top the salmon with lemon slices and bake for 15-20 minutes, until the salmon is cooked through and the asparagus is tender.
- Serve with a side of cooked quinoa for a complete, nutrient-rich meal that supports hormonal health.

Nutritional Information (per serving):

- Calories: 450 kcal
- Protein: 35g
- Fat: 20g
- Carbohydrates: 25g
- Fiber: 5g
- Omega-3: 2g
- Vitamin C: 30% RDA

Nutritional Benefits:

Salmon is rich in omega-3 fatty acids, which help regulate hormone production and reduce inflammation. Asparagus is high in folate and antioxidants, and quinoa provides a complete source of protein, making this a balanced and hormone-supportive dinner.

Turkey and Zucchini Meatballs with Tomato Sauce

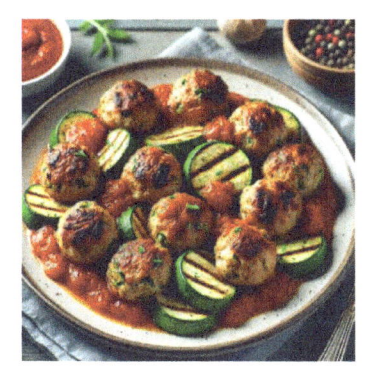

Servings: 1

Cooking Time: 35 minutes

Ingredients:

- 1 pound ground turkey
- 1 zucchini, grated
- 1 egg
- 1/4 cup breadcrumbs (or almond flour for gluten-free)
- 2 garlic cloves, minced
- 1 tablespoon fresh parsley, chopped
- 1 jar (16 oz) tomato sauce (low-sodium)
- 1 tablespoon olive oil
- Salt and pepper to taste

Instructions:

- Preheat your oven to 400°F (200°C). In a large bowl, combine the ground turkey, grated zucchini, egg, breadcrumbs, garlic, parsley, salt, and pepper.
- Roll the mixture into small meatballs and place them on a baking sheet.
- Bake for 15-20 minutes, until the meatballs are cooked through.
- In a saucepan, heat the tomato sauce over medium heat. Add the meatballs to the sauce and simmer for 5 minutes.
- Serve over whole-grain pasta or spaghetti squash for a hearty, hormone-supportive dinner.

Nutritional Information (per serving):

- Calories: 350 kcal
- Protein: 28g
- Fat: 12g
- Carbohydrates: 30g
- Fiber: 8g
- Iron: 15% RDA
- Vitamin C: 25% RDA

Nutritional Benefits:

Turkey is a lean protein that helps regulate blood sugar and supports muscle repair, important for maintaining hormonal balance. Zucchini adds fiber and antioxidants, while tomatoes are rich in lycopene, a powerful antioxidant that reduces oxidative stress.

Lentil and Sweet Potato Curry

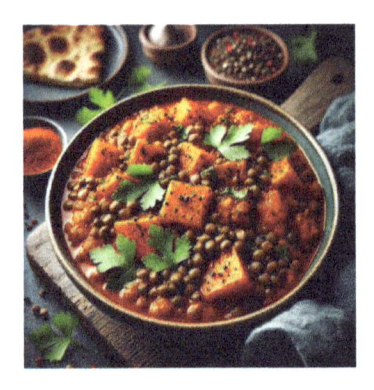

Servings: 1

Cooking Time: 40 minutes

Ingredients:

- 1 cup dried lentils, rinsed
- 1 sweet potato, peeled and diced
- 1 onion, diced
- 2 garlic cloves, minced
- 1 tablespoon curry powder
- 1 can (14 oz) coconut milk
- 2 cups vegetable broth
- 1 tablespoon olive oil
- Salt and pepper to taste

Instructions:

- Heat the olive oil in a large pot over medium heat. Add the onion and garlic, and sauté until softened.
- Add the curry powder and stir for 1 minute to release the flavors.
- Stir in the lentils, sweet potato, coconut milk, and vegetable broth. Bring to a boil, then reduce the heat and simmer for 25-30 minutes, until the lentils and sweet potatoes are tender.
- Season with salt and pepper, and serve with brown rice or naan bread for a satisfying, hormone-supportive dinner.

Nutritional Information (per serving):

- Calories: 400 kcal
- Protein: 14g
- Fat: 18g
- Carbohydrates: 48g
- Fiber: 12g
- Iron: 20% RDA
- Vitamin A: 200% RDA

Nutritional Benefits:

Lentils are a great source of plant-based protein, iron, and fiber, all of which support healthy ovulation and hormonal balance. Sweet potatoes are rich in beta-carotene, which aids in the production of progesterone, a key hormone in fertility.

Grilled Chicken with Roasted Vegetables

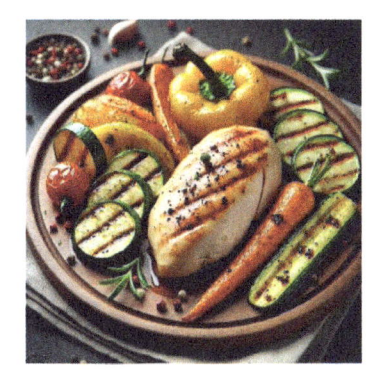

Servings: 1

Cooking Time: 30 minutes

Ingredients:

- 2 chicken breasts
- 1 red bell pepper, sliced
- 1 zucchini, sliced
- 1 carrot, peeled and sliced
- 2 tablespoons olive oil
- 1 teaspoon dried oregano
- Salt and pepper to taste

Instructions:

- Preheat your grill to medium-high heat. Season the chicken breasts with olive oil, oregano, salt, and pepper.
- Grill the chicken for 5-6 minutes per side, until fully cooked.
- In a separate pan, toss the bell pepper, zucchini, and carrot with olive oil, salt, and pepper. Roast in the oven at 400°F (200°C) for 20-25 minutes, until tender.
- Serve the grilled chicken alongside the roasted vegetables for a balanced, nutrient-packed dinner that supports hormonal health.

Nutritional Information (per serving):

- Calories: 400 kcal
- Protein: 35g
- Fat: 18g
- Carbohydrates: 15g
- Fiber: 6g
- Vitamin C: 100% RDA
- Iron: 10% RDA

Nutritional Benefits:

Grilled chicken provides lean protein, which helps balance blood sugar and supports muscle repair, while roasted vegetables like bell peppers and carrots are rich in antioxidants and fiber, aiding in hormonal balance and digestion.

Cod with Spinach and White Beans

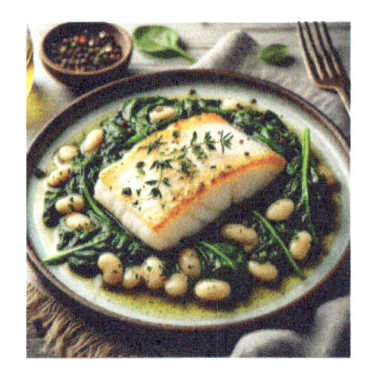

Servings: 1

Cooking Time: 20 minutes

Ingredients:

- 2 cod fillets
- 2 cups fresh spinach
- 1 can (15 oz) white beans, drained and rinsed
- 1 garlic clove, minced
- 1 tablespoon olive oil
- 1 tablespoon lemon juice
- Salt and pepper to taste

Instructions:

- Heat the olive oil in a large skillet over medium heat. Add the garlic and cook for 1 minute until fragrant.
- Add the cod fillets to the skillet and cook for 3-4 minutes on each side until the fish is opaque and flakes easily with a fork.
- In a separate pan, sauté the spinach until wilted, then stir in the white beans and lemon juice.
- Serve the cod over the spinach and beans for a light, protein-rich dinner that supports hormonal health and fertility.

Nutritional Information (per serving):

- Calories: 350 kcal
- Protein: 32g
- Fat: 10g
- Carbohydrates: 28g
- Fiber: 8g
- Vitamin C: 20% RDA
- Iron: 20% RDA

Nutritional Benefits:

Cod is a lean, high-protein fish that is low in fat and provides key nutrients like selenium, which supports thyroid function and hormone production. Spinach is rich in folate and iron, and white beans provide fiber and plant-based protein for hormonal balance.

Eggplant and Chickpea Stew

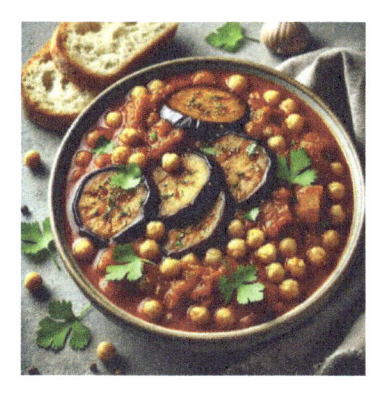

Servings: 1

Cooking Time: 35 minutes

Ingredients:

- 1 large eggplant, diced
- 1 can (15 oz) chickpeas, drained and rinsed
- 1 onion, diced
- 2 garlic cloves, minced
- 1 teaspoon cumin
- 1 teaspoon paprika
- 1 can (14 oz) diced tomatoes
- 1 tablespoon olive oil
- Salt and pepper to taste

Instructions:

- Heat the olive oil in a large pot over medium heat. Add the onion and garlic, and sauté until softened.
- Stir in the cumin and paprika, and cook for 1 minute to release the flavors.
- Add the diced eggplant, chickpeas, and diced tomatoes. Bring to a boil, then reduce the heat and simmer for 20-25 minutes, until the eggplant is tender.
- Season with salt and pepper, and serve over brown rice or with crusty bread for a filling, hormone-supportive dinner.

Nutritional Information (per serving):

- Calories: 300 kcal
- Protein: 10g
- Fat: 12g
- Carbohydrates: 40g
- Fiber: 10g
- Iron: 15% RDA
- Vitamin A: 15% RDA

Nutritional Benefits:

Eggplant is high in fiber and antioxidants, while chickpeas provide plant-based protein and folate, which support hormonal health and reproductive function. This hearty stew is also rich in anti-inflammatory spices that help reduce oxidative stress.

Shrimp Stir-Fry with Broccoli and Cashews

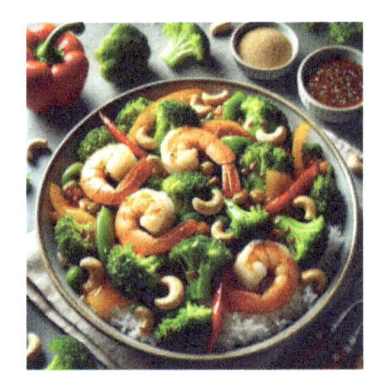

Servings: 1

Cooking Time: 15 minutes

Ingredients:

- 1/2-pound shrimp, peeled and deveined
- 1 cup broccoli florets
- 1/4 cup cashews, chopped
- 1 garlic clove, minced
- 1 tablespoon soy sauce (or tamari for gluten-free)
- 1 tablespoon sesame oil
- Salt and pepper to taste

Instructions:

- Heat the sesame oil in a large skillet over medium heat. Add the garlic and cook until fragrant.
- Add the shrimp and broccoli to the skillet, and stir-fry for 5-7 minutes until the shrimp is pink and the broccoli is tender.
- Stir in the soy sauce and cashews, and cook for another 2 minutes.
- Serve hot for a quick, protein-rich dinner that supports hormone balance and overall reproductive health.

Nutritional Information (per serving):

- Calories: 350 kcal
- Protein: 28g
- Fat: 18g
- Carbohydrates: 12g
- Fiber: 4g
- Omega-3: 1g
- Iron: 15% RDA

Nutritional Benefits:

Shrimp is a low-fat source of protein and selenium, which plays a key role in thyroid function and reproductive health. Broccoli is rich in fiber and antioxidants, while cashews add healthy fats and zinc, both important for hormonal balance.

Chicken and Sweet Potato Bake

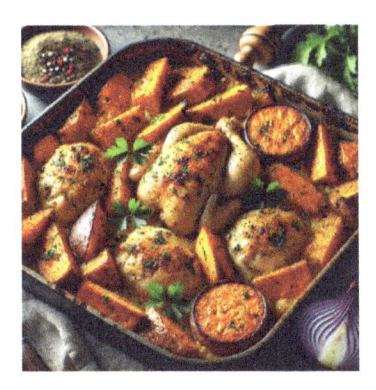

Servings: 1

Cooking Time: 40 minutes

Ingredients:

- 2 chicken thighs, bone-in, skin removed
- 2 medium sweet potatoes, peeled and diced
- 1 red onion, sliced
- 2 tablespoons olive oil
- 1 teaspoon rosemary
- Salt and pepper to taste

Instructions:

- Preheat the oven to 375°F (190°C). Place the chicken thighs, sweet potatoes, and onion in a baking dish.
- Drizzle with olive oil, sprinkle with rosemary, and season with salt and pepper.
- Bake for 35-40 minutes, until the chicken is cooked through and the sweet potatoes are tender.
- Serve hot for a nourishing, hormone-supportive dinner that balances protein and healthy carbohydrates.

Nutritional Information (per serving):

- Calories: 500 kcal
- Protein: 35g
- Fat: 20g
- Carbohydrates: 45g
- Fiber: 8g
- Vitamin A: 200% RDA
- Iron: 15% RDA

Nutritional Benefits:

Chicken provides lean protein that supports muscle repair and hormonal balance, while sweet potatoes are rich in beta-carotene and fiber, which aid in progesterone production and support overall reproductive health.

Quinoa-Stuffed Bell Peppers

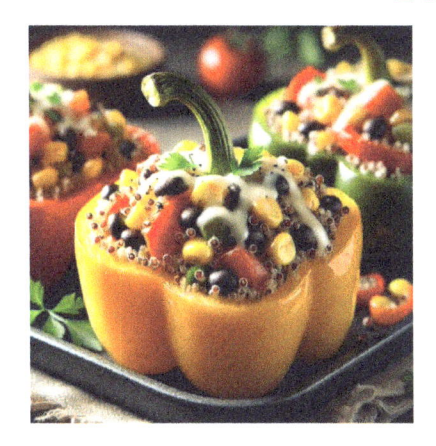

Servings: 1

Cooking Time: 35 minutes

Ingredients:

- 4 large bell peppers, tops cut off and seeds removed
- 1 cup cooked quinoa
- 1/2 cup black beans, cooked
- 1/4 cup corn kernels
- 1 tablespoon olive oil
- 1 teaspoon cumin
- Salt and pepper to taste

Instructions:

- Preheat your oven to 375°F (190°C). In a large bowl, combine the cooked quinoa, black beans, corn, olive oil, cumin, salt, and pepper.
- Stuff the mixture into the prepared bell peppers and place them in a baking dish.
- Cover the dish with foil and bake for 25-30 minutes, until the peppers are tender.
- Serve hot for a hearty, plant-based dinner that supports hormonal health and fertility.

Nutritional Information (per serving):

- Calories: 350 kcal
- Protein: 12g
- Fat: 12g
- Carbohydrates: 48g
- Fiber: 10g
- Vitamin C: 200% RDA
- Folate: 30% RDA

Nutritional Benefits:

Quinoa is a complete protein and provides a rich source of magnesium, important for regulating stress and supporting hormonal balance. Bell peppers are high in vitamin C and antioxidants, while black beans add fiber and plant-based protein to this filling dish.

Grilled Tofu with Roasted Brussels Sprouts

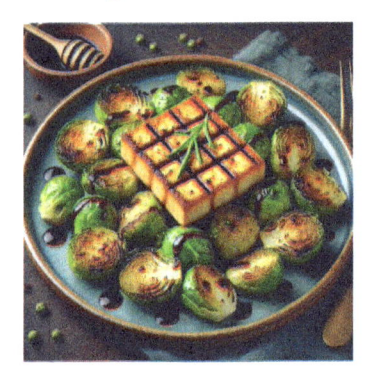

Servings: 1
Cooking Time: 30 minutes

Ingredients:

- 1 block firm tofu, drained and sliced
- 2 cups Brussels sprouts, halved
- 2 tablespoons olive oil
- 1 tablespoon soy sauce (or tamari for gluten-free)
- 1 garlic clove, minced
- Salt and pepper to taste

Instructions:

- Preheat your oven to 400°F (200°C). Toss the Brussels sprouts with olive oil, garlic, salt, and pepper. Spread them on a baking sheet and roast for 20-25 minutes, until crispy.
- While the Brussels sprouts are roasting, heat a grill pan over medium heat. Brush the tofu slices with soy sauce and grill for 3-4 minutes on each side until golden brown.
- Serve the grilled tofu alongside the roasted Brussels sprouts for a balanced, protein-rich dinner that supports hormonal health.

Nutritional Benefits:

Tofu is a great plant-based source of protein and contains phytoestrogens that help balance hormone levels. Brussels sprouts are rich in fiber, antioxidants, and vitamins that support reproductive health and digestion.

CHAPTER 5

SNACKS AND DESSERTS RECIPES

Almond and Chia Seed Energy Bites

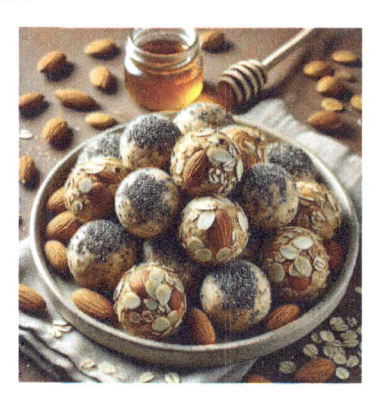

Servings: 1

Cooking Time: 10 minutes (plus 30 minutes to chill)

Ingredients:

- 1 cup rolled oats
- 1/2 cup almond butter
- 1/4 cup chia seeds
- 1/4 cup honey or maple syrup
- 1/4 cup dark chocolate chips (optional)
- 1 teaspoon vanilla extract

Instructions:

- In a large bowl, combine all ingredients and mix until well combined.

- Roll the mixture into small bite-sized balls and place them on a baking sheet.
- Refrigerate for at least 30 minutes to firm up.
- Store the energy bites in an airtight container in the fridge for up to a week for a quick and satisfying snack.

Nutritional Information (per bite):

- Calories: 100 kcal
- Protein: 3g
- Fat: 6g
- Carbohydrates: 10g
- Fiber: 3g
- Omega-3: 1.5g
- Iron: 5% RDA

Nutritional Benefits:

Almonds are rich in vitamin E, which supports egg quality, and chia seeds provide a powerful dose of omega-3 fatty acids and fiber. These energy bites are a perfect portable snack that helps balance blood sugar and keep you feeling full.

Greek Yogurt with Pumpkin Seeds and Berries

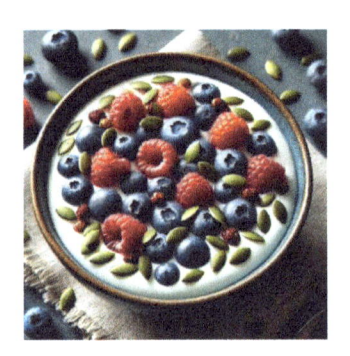

Servings: 1
Cooking Time: 5 minutes

Ingredients:

- 1/2 cup plain Greek yogurt (or a dairy-free alternative)
- 2 tablespoons pumpkin seeds
- 1/4 cup mixed berries (blueberries, raspberries, etc.)
- 1 teaspoon honey or maple syrup (optional)

Instructions:

- In a small bowl, layer the Greek yogurt, pumpkin seeds, and berries.
- Drizzle with honey or maple syrup if desired.
- Enjoy a nutrient-rich snack that supports fertility and provides a good balance of protein, healthy fats, and antioxidants.

Nutritional Information (per serving):

- Calories: 200 kcal

- Protein: 12g
- Fat: 8g
- Carbohydrates: 20g
- Fiber: 4g
- Calcium: 15% RDA
- Vitamin C: 10% RDA

Nutritional Benefits:

Greek yogurt is a great source of protein and probiotics, which support gut health and hormone regulation. Pumpkin seeds provide zinc and healthy fats, while berries are loaded with antioxidants, making this snack both refreshing and fertility-boosting.

Roasted Chickpeas with Spices

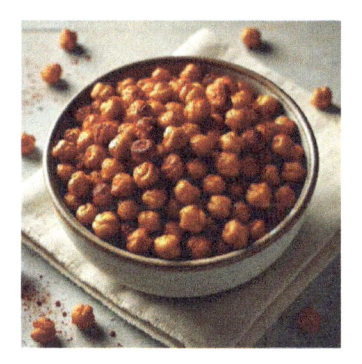

Servings: 4

Cooking Time: 30 minutes

Ingredients:

- 1 can (15 oz) chickpeas, drained and rinsed
- 1 tablespoon olive oil
- 1 teaspoon cumin
- 1/2 teaspoon paprika
- Salt and pepper to taste

Instructions:

- Preheat your oven to 400°F (200°C). Pat the chickpeas dry with a paper towel and spread them on a baking sheet.
- Drizzle with olive oil, sprinkle with spices, and toss to coat evenly.
- Roast for 25-30 minutes, shaking the pan halfway through, until the chickpeas are crispy and golden brown.
- Let cool before serving. Store in an airtight container for a quick, crunchy snack that supports fertility.

Nutritional Information (per serving):

- Calories: 180 kcal
- Protein: 6g
- Fat: 6g
- Carbohydrates: 25g
- Fiber: 7g
- Iron: 10% RDA
- Folate: 15% RDA

Nutritional Benefits:

Chickpeas are rich in plant-based protein, fiber, and folate, all of which are essential for reproductive health. Roasting them with spices creates a crunchy, savory snack that's perfect for satisfying cravings in a healthy way.

Apple Slices with Almond Butter

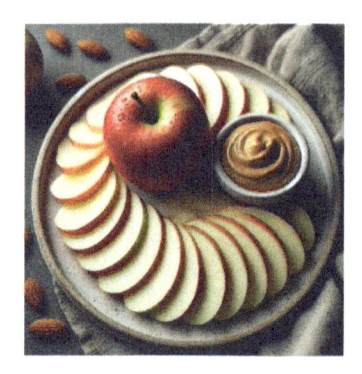

Servings: 1

Cooking Time: 5 minutes

Ingredients:

- 1 apple, sliced
- 2 tablespoons almond butter
- A sprinkle of cinnamon (optional)

Instructions:

- Slice the apple and arrange the slices on a plate.
- Spread almond butter on each slice and sprinkle with cinnamon if desired.
- Enjoy a crunchy, satisfying snack that's rich in fiber, healthy fats, and fertility-supporting nutrients.

Nutritional Information (per serving):

- Calories: 250 kcal
- Protein: 4g
- Fat: 12g
- Carbohydrates: 34g
- Fiber: 7g
- Vitamin C: 15% RDA
- Calcium: 4% RDA

Nutritional Benefits:

Apples are a great source of fiber, while almond butter provides healthy fats and protein, making this snack a simple yet effective way to keep blood sugar stable and promote hormonal balance.

Hard-Boiled Eggs with Avocado

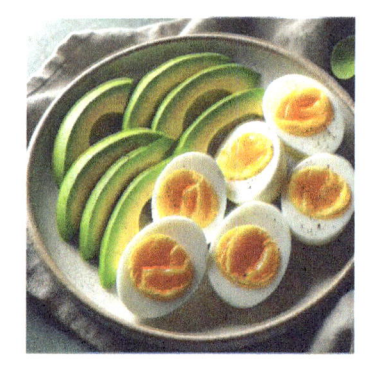

Servings: 1

Cooking Time: 10 minutes

Ingredients:

- 2 hard-boiled eggs
- 1/2 avocado, sliced
- Salt and pepper to taste

Instructions:

- Peel and slice the hard-boiled eggs.
- Arrange the egg slices on a plate and top with avocado slices.
- Season with salt and pepper, and enjoy a protein-rich, hormone-supporting snack.

Nutritional Information (per serving):

- Calories: 260 kcal
- Protein: 12g
- Fat: 22g
- Carbohydrates: 6g
- Fiber: 5g
- Vitamin D: 15% RDA
- Potassium: 10% RDA

Nutritional Benefits:

Eggs are a powerhouse of protein and essential nutrients like choline and vitamin D, both of which support fertility and hormonal balance. Pairing eggs with avocado, which is rich in healthy fats, makes this a satiating and nutrient-packed snack.

Trail Mix with Walnuts, Dark Chocolate, and Dried Fruit

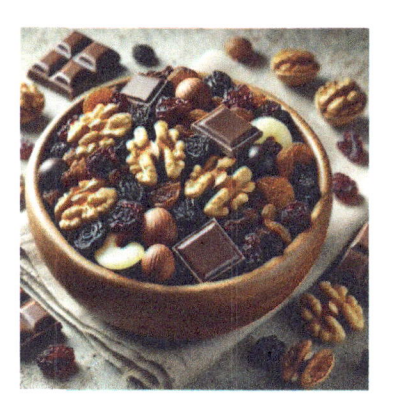

Servings: 1

Cooking Time: 5 minutes

Ingredients:

- 1/4 cup walnuts
- 1/4 cup dark chocolate chips
- 1/4 cup dried cranberries or raisins
- 1/4 cup almonds or cashews

Instructions:

- Combine all ingredients in a bowl and mix well.
- Store in an airtight container for a quick, portable snack that satisfies cravings and provides fertility-boosting nutrients.

Nutritional Information (per serving):

- Calories: 150 kcal
- Protein: 4g

- Fat: 8g
- Carbohydrates: 15g
- Fiber: 5g
- Calcium: 6% RDA
- Iron: 8% RDA

Nutritional Benefits:

Walnuts are rich in omega-3 fatty acids, which are essential for reducing inflammation and supporting fertility. Dark chocolate provides antioxidants, and dried fruit adds natural sweetness, making this a satisfying snack that also supports reproductive health.

Celery Sticks with Hummus

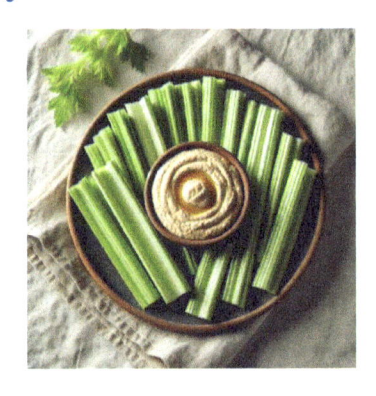

Servings: 1

Cooking Time: 5 minutes

Ingredients:

- 4 celery stalks, cut into sticks
- 1/4 cup hummus

Instructions:

- Arrange the celery sticks on a plate and serve with a side of hummus for dipping.
- Enjoy a crunchy, fiber-rich snack that helps maintain energy levels and supports fertility.

Nutritional Information (per serving):

- Calories: 150 kcal
- Protein: 12g
- Fat: 5g
- Carbohydrates: 15g
- Fiber: 2g
- Vitamin C: 10% RDA
- Calcium: 12% RDA

Nutritional Benefits:

Celery is low in calories but high in fiber, making it a great snack for keeping you full between meals. Hummus, made from chickpeas, is rich in protein, fiber, and healthy fats, supporting hormonal balance and reproductive health.

Cottage Cheese with Pineapple

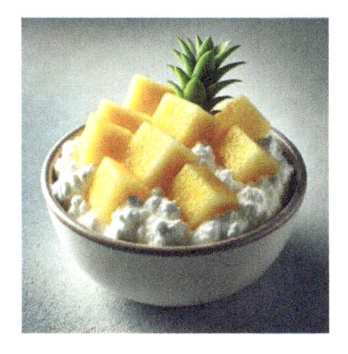

Servings: 1

Cooking Time: 5 minutes

Ingredients:

- 1/2 cup cottage cheese (or a dairy-free alternative)
- 1/4 cup fresh pineapple chunks

Instructions:

- In a small bowl, combine the cottage cheese and pineapple.
- Serve chilled for a refreshing, protein-packed snack that supports fertility and digestion.

Nutritional Information (per serving):

- Calories: 150 kcal
- Protein: 12g
- Fat: 5g
- Carbohydrates: 15g
- Fiber: 2g
- Vitamin C: 10% RDA
- Calcium: 12% RDA

Nutritional Benefits:

Cottage cheese is an excellent source of protein and calcium, both of which are important for hormone regulation and bone health. Pineapple adds a burst of sweetness and is rich in bromelain, an enzyme that can support implantation and reproductive health.

Carrot and Cucumber Sticks with Tahini Dip

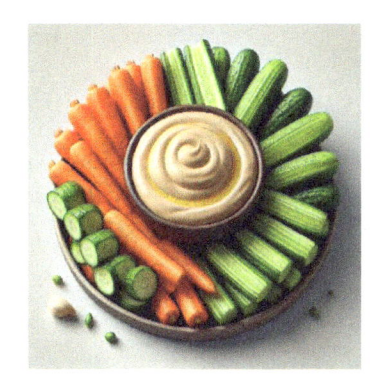

Servings: 1

Cooking Time: 5 minutes

Ingredients:

- 2 carrots, peeled and cut into sticks
- 1 cucumber, sliced into sticks
- 2 tablespoons tahini
- 1 tablespoon lemon juice
- Salt and pepper to taste

Instructions:

- In a small bowl, whisk together the tahini, lemon juice, salt, and pepper to make the dip.
- Serve the carrot and cucumber sticks alongside the tahini dip for a crunchy, nutrient-dense snack that's perfect for fertility support.

Nutritional Information (per serving):

- Calories: 200 kcal
- Protein: 6g
- Fat: 15g
- Carbohydrates: 16g
- Fiber: 6g
- Vitamin A: 150% RDA
- Iron: 10% RDA

Nutritional Benefits:

Carrots and cucumbers are rich in fiber and antioxidants, while tahini (made from sesame seeds) provides healthy fats and calcium, both of which support hormonal balance and overall fertility.

Banana and Peanut Butter Smoothie

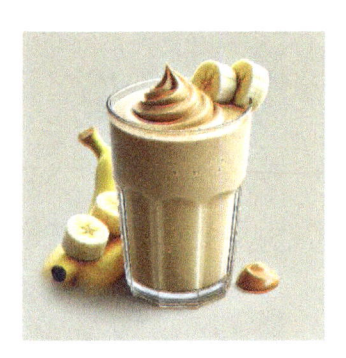

Servings: 1

Cooking Time: 5 minutes

Ingredients:

- 1 ripe banana
- 1 tablespoon peanut butter
- 1/2 cup unsweetened almond milk
- 1/4 teaspoon cinnamon
- Ice cubes (optional)

Instructions:

- In a blender, combine the banana, peanut butter, almond milk, cinnamon, and ice cubes if desired.
- Blend until smooth and creamy.
- Serve immediately for a refreshing, protein-packed snack that supports energy levels and fertility.

Nutritional Information (per serving):

- Calories: 250 kcal
- Protein: 6g
- Fat: 12g
- Carbohydrates: 34g
- Fiber: 5g
- Potassium: 20% RDA
- Vitamin B6: 30% RDA

Nutritional Benefits:

Bananas are rich in potassium and vitamin B6, both of which help regulate hormone production. Peanut butter provides healthy fats and protein, making this smoothie a satisfying and fertility-friendly snack.

Dark Chocolate Avocado Mousse

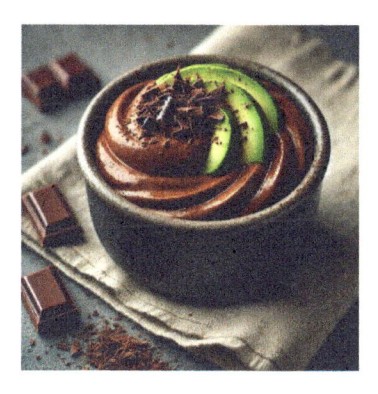

Servings: 1

Cooking Time: 10 minutes (plus 30 minutes chilling time)

Ingredients:

- 2 ripe avocados
- 1/4 cup unsweetened cocoa powder
- 1/4 cup maple syrup or honey
- 1 teaspoon vanilla extract
- A pinch of sea salt
- Fresh berries for topping (optional)

Instructions:

- In a blender or food processor, combine the avocados, cocoa powder, maple syrup, vanilla extract, and sea salt. Blend until smooth and creamy.
- Transfer the mousse to small bowls and refrigerate for at least 30 minutes to allow it to set.
- Serve chilled with fresh berries for a decadent, fertility-boosting dessert.

Nutritional Information (per serving):

- Calories: 250 kcal
- Protein: 3g
- Fat: 18g
- Carbohydrates: 26g
- Fiber: 8g
- Potassium: 15% RDA
- Iron: 10% RDA

Nutritional Benefits:

Dark chocolate is rich in antioxidants, which help protect cells from oxidative stress, while avocado provides healthy fats that support hormonal balance. This mousse is creamy, indulgent, and packed with nutrients.

Baked Apples with Cinnamon and Walnuts

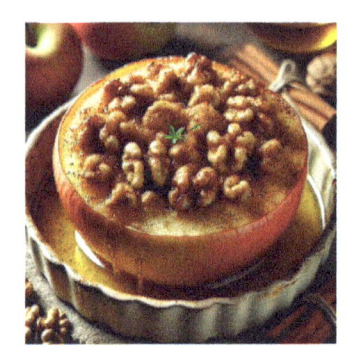

Servings: 1

Cooking Time: 30 minutes

Ingredients:

- 4 medium apples, cored
- 1/4 cup walnuts, chopped
- 1 tablespoon honey or maple syrup
- 1 teaspoon ground cinnamon
- 1 tablespoon coconut oil

Instructions:

- Preheat your oven to 350°F (175°C).
- Place the cored apples in a baking dish. In a small bowl, combine the chopped walnuts, honey, cinnamon, and coconut oil.
- Stuff the walnut mixture into the center of each apple.
- Bake for 25-30 minutes, until the apples are tender.
- Serve warm for a comforting, nutrient-rich dessert that supports hormonal balance.

Nutritional Information (per serving):

- Calories: 200 kcal
- Protein: 2g
- Fat: 8g
- Carbohydrates: 32g
- Fiber: 6g
- Vitamin C: 10% RDA
- Omega-3: 0.5g

Nutritional Benefits:

Apples are a great source of fiber and antioxidants, while cinnamon helps regulate blood sugar levels. Walnuts add omega-3 fatty acids, which reduce inflammation and support fertility.

Chia Pudding with Coconut and Mango

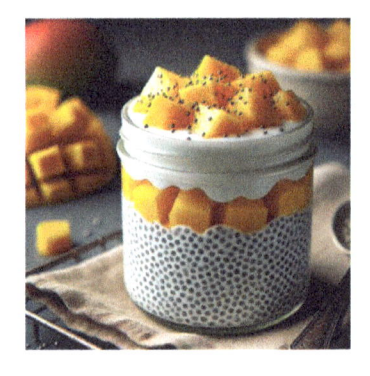

Servings: 1

Cooking Time: 10 minutes (plus 4 hours chilling time)

Ingredients:

- 1/4 cup chia seeds
- 1 cup unsweetened coconut milk
- 1 teaspoon vanilla extract
- 1 tablespoon honey or maple syrup (optional)
- 1/2 cup fresh or frozen mango, diced
- 1 tablespoon shredded coconut for garnish

Instructions:

- In a jar or bowl, combine the chia seeds, coconut milk, vanilla extract, and honey or maple syrup.
- Stir well, cover, and refrigerate for at least 4 hours, or overnight, to allow the chia seeds to thicken.
- Before serving, top with diced mango and shredded coconut for a tropical, fertility-friendly dessert.

Nutritional Information (per serving):

- Calories: 240 kcal
- Protein: 6g
- Fat: 12g
- Carbohydrates: 32g
- Fiber: 10g
- Omega-3: 3g
- Vitamin C: 20% RDA

Nutritional Benefits:

Chia seeds are loaded with omega-3 fatty acids and fiber, which help balance hormones and support digestion. Coconut adds healthy fats, and mango provides natural sweetness and a dose of vitamin C, which is important for reproductive health.

Almond Flour Brownies

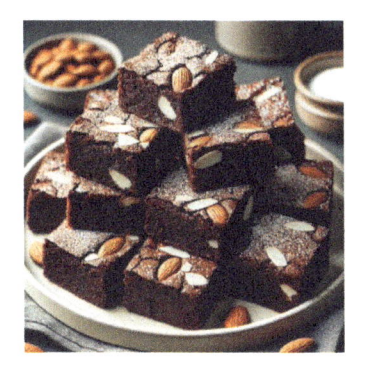

Servings: 1

Cooking Time: 25 minutes

Ingredients:

- 1 cup almond flour
- 1/4 cup unsweetened cocoa powder
- 1/4 cup maple syrup or honey
- 1/4 cup coconut oil, melted
- 2 eggs
- 1 teaspoon vanilla extract
- 1/2 teaspoon baking soda
- A pinch of sea salt

Instructions:

- Preheat your oven to 350°F (175°C) and grease a small baking pan with coconut oil.
- In a large bowl, whisk together the almond flour, cocoa powder, baking soda, and sea salt.
- In a separate bowl, combine the eggs, coconut oil, maple syrup, and vanilla extract.
- Pour the wet ingredients into the dry ingredients and mix until well combined.
- Pour the batter into the greased baking pan and bake for 20-25 minutes, until a toothpick comes out clean.
- Allow the brownies to cool before slicing. Serve for a rich, fertility-boosting dessert.

Nutritional Information (per serving):

- Calories: 180 kcal
- Protein: 5g
- Fat: 14g
- Carbohydrates: 12g
- Fiber: 4g
- Vitamin E: 20% RDA
- Iron: 8% RDA

Nutritional Benefits:

Almond flour is a great alternative to refined flour, as it's rich in vitamin E and healthy fats that support reproductive health. These brownies are naturally sweetened and gluten-free, making them a perfect treat for IVF mothers.

Berry Crumble with Oats and Almonds

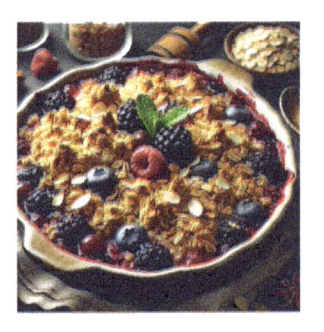

Servings: 1

Cooking Time: 25 minutes

Ingredients:

- 2 cups mixed berries (blueberries, raspberries, strawberries)
- 1/2 cup rolled oats
- 1/4 cup almond flour
- 1/4 cup sliced almonds
- 2 tablespoons coconut oil, melted
- 1 tablespoon honey or maple syrup
- 1 teaspoon cinnamon

Instructions:

- Preheat your oven to 350°F (175°C). In a baking dish, spread the mixed berries evenly.
- In a small bowl, combine the oats, almond flour, sliced almonds, coconut oil, honey, and cinnamon.

- Sprinkle the oat mixture over the berries.
- Bake for 20-25 minutes, until the topping is golden and the berries are bubbling.
- Serve warm for a comforting, antioxidant-rich dessert that supports fertility.

Nutritional Information (per serving):

- Calories: 240 kcal
- Protein: 4g
- Fat: 14g
- Carbohydrates: 28g
- Fiber: 7g
- Vitamin C: 20% RDA
- Iron: 8% RDA

Nutritional Benefits:

Berries are packed with antioxidants, which help protect eggs from oxidative stress. Oats provide fiber for digestion, while almonds add healthy fats and protein, making this crumble a nourishing dessert.

Coconut Macaroons

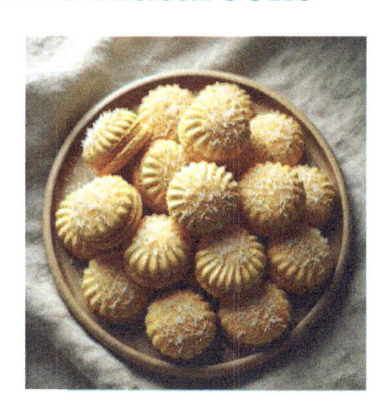

Servings: 1

Cooking Time: 20 minutes

Ingredients:

- 2 cups shredded unsweetened coconut
- 1/4 cup maple syrup or honey
- 2 egg whites
- 1 teaspoon vanilla extract
- A pinch of sea salt

Instructions:

- Preheat your oven to 325°F (160°C) and line a baking sheet with parchment paper.
- In a large bowl, whisk the egg whites until frothy.
- Stir in the shredded coconut, maple syrup, vanilla extract, and sea salt.
- Scoop tablespoon-sized portions of the mixture onto the prepared baking sheet.
- Bake for 15-20 minutes, until the edges are golden.

- Allow the macaroons to cool before serving for a light, nutrient-rich dessert.

Nutritional Information (per macaroon):

- Calories: 100 kcal
- Protein: 2g
- Fat: 7g
- Carbohydrates: 8g
- Fiber: 2g
- Iron: 4% RDA
- Calcium: 2% RDA

Nutritional Benefits:

Coconut is rich in healthy fats that support hormone production, while these macaroons are naturally sweetened and free from refined sugars, making them a guilt-free treat for IVF mothers.

Chocolate-Covered Strawberries

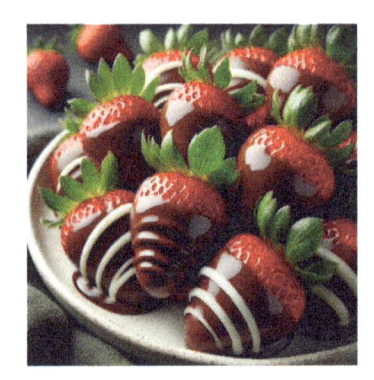

Servings: 1

Cooking Time: 15 minutes

Ingredients:

- 1 cup fresh strawberries
- 1/2 cup dark chocolate chips (70% cacao or higher)
- 1 tablespoon coconut oil

Instructions:

- Wash and dry the strawberries thoroughly.
- In a small saucepan, melt the dark chocolate and coconut oil over low heat, stirring until smooth.
- Dip each strawberry into the melted chocolate and place them on a parchment-lined baking sheet.
- Refrigerate for 10-15 minutes, or until the chocolate is set.
- Serve chilled for a delicious, antioxidant-packed dessert.

Nutritional Information (per serving):

- Calories: 150 kcal
- Protein: 1g
- Fat: 10g
- Carbohydrates: 18g
- Fiber: 4g
- Vitamin C: 80% RDA
- Iron: 10% RDA

Nutritional Benefits:

Strawberries are rich in vitamin C and antioxidants, while dark chocolate provides a dose of healthy fats and minerals that support fertility. This simple, elegant dessert is perfect for satisfying sweet cravings while nourishing your body.

Lemon and Blueberry Greek Yogurt Popsicles

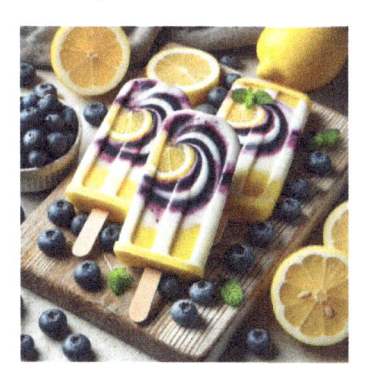

Servings: 4 popsicles

Cooking Time: 5 minutes (plus 4 hours freezing time)

Ingredients:

- 1 cup plain Greek yogurt
- 1/4 cup fresh blueberries
- 2 tablespoons lemon juice
- 2 tablespoons honey or maple syrup

Instructions:

- In a blender, combine the Greek yogurt, lemon juice, and honey or maple syrup until smooth.
- Stir in the fresh blueberries.
- Pour the mixture into popsicle molds and freeze for at least 4 hours, or until solid.
- Enjoy these creamy, antioxidant-rich popsicles as a cool, fertility-friendly dessert.

Nutritional Information (per popsicle):

- Calories: 100 kcal
- Protein: 5g
- Fat: 1g
- Carbohydrates: 18g
- Fiber: 1g
- Calcium: 10% RDA
- Vitamin C: 10% RDA

Nutritional Benefits:

Greek yogurt provides probiotics and protein, while blueberries are rich in antioxidants that protect egg health. These refreshing popsicles are a perfect summer treat that supports fertility.

No-Bake Peanut Butter Bars

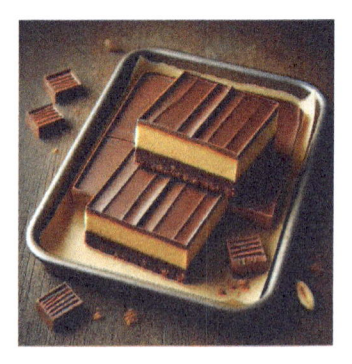

Servings: 1

Cooking Time: 10 minutes (plus 1 hour chilling time)

Ingredients:

- 1 cup rolled oats
- 1/2 cup natural peanut butter
- 1/4 cup honey or maple syrup
- 1/4 cup dark chocolate chips (optional)
- 1 teaspoon vanilla extract

Instructions:

- In a large bowl, combine the oats, peanut butter, honey, and vanilla extract. Mix until well combined.
- Press the mixture into a lined baking dish and refrigerate for at least 1 hour.
- Melt the dark chocolate chips (if using) and drizzle over the top.
- Slice into bars and serve for a quick, no-bake dessert that satisfies your sweet cravings while supporting fertility.

Nutritional Information (per bar):

- Calories: 220 kcal
- Protein: 6g
- Fat: 12g
- Carbohydrates: 22g
- Fiber: 4g
- Iron: 6% RDA
- Calcium: 4% RDA

Nutritional Benefits:

Peanut butter is a great source of healthy fats and protein, while oats provide fiber and slow-digesting carbohydrates. These no-bake bars are naturally sweetened and make a satisfying, energy-boosting dessert.

Banana Nice Cream

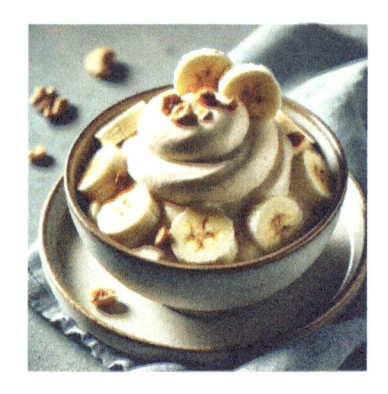

Servings: 1

Cooking Time: 5 minutes

Ingredients:

- 2 ripe bananas, sliced and frozen
- 1/2 teaspoon vanilla extract

- 1 tablespoon almond butter (optional)
- 1/4 cup almond milk

Instructions:

- In a food processor or blender, combine the frozen banana slices, vanilla extract, almond butter (if using), and almond milk.
- Blend until smooth and creamy, scraping down the sides as needed.
- Serve immediately for a refreshing, fertility-friendly ice cream alternative.

Nutritional Information (per serving):

- Calories: 150 kcal
- Protein: 2g
- Fat: 4g
- Carbohydrates: 30g
- Fiber: 4g
- Potassium: 20% RDA
- Vitamin B6: 30% RDA

Nutritional Benefits:

Bananas are rich in potassium and vitamin B6, both of which help regulate hormones. This dairy-free "nice cream" is a creamy, naturally sweet treat that's perfect for a healthy dessert.

CHAPTER 6

SOUP AND STEW RECIPES

Lentil and Vegetable Soup

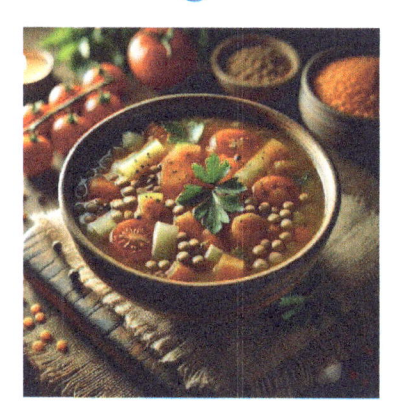

Servings: 1

Cooking Time: 35 minutes

Ingredients:

- 1 cup dried lentils, rinsed
- 1 onion, diced
- 2 carrots, diced
- 2 celery stalks, chopped
- 3 garlic cloves, minced
- 1 can (14.5 oz) diced tomatoes
- 4 cups vegetable broth
- 1 tablespoon olive oil
- 1 teaspoon cumin
- 1 teaspoon thyme
- Salt and pepper to taste

Instructions:

- Heat olive oil in a large pot over medium heat. Sauté onion, carrots, celery, and garlic until softened, about 5 minutes.
- Add lentils, diced tomatoes, vegetable broth, cumin, and thyme. Bring to a boil.
- Reduce heat, cover, and simmer for 25-30 minutes, until lentils are tender.
- Season with salt and pepper to taste and serve.

Nutritional Benefits:

Lentils are rich in protein, fiber, and folate, supporting hormone regulation and digestion, both of which are crucial for reproductive health.

Nutritional Information (per serving):

- Calories: 250 kcal
- Protein: 12g
- Fat: 4g
- Carbohydrates: 38g
- Fiber: 12g
- Iron: 20% RDA
- Folate: 50% RDA

Chicken and Sweet Potato Stew

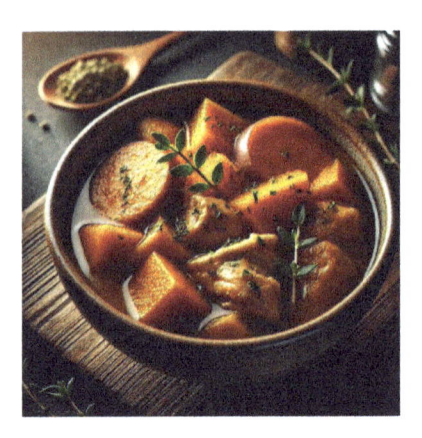

Servings: 1

Cooking Time: 40 minutes

Ingredients:

- 2 chicken breasts, diced
- 2 sweet potatoes, peeled and diced
- 1 onion, chopped
- 2 garlic cloves, minced
- 4 cups chicken broth
- 1 cup spinach
- 1 tablespoon olive oil
- 1 teaspoon paprika
- 1/2 teaspoon cayenne pepper (optional)
- Salt and pepper to taste

Instructions:

- Heat olive oil in a pot over medium heat. Sauté onion and garlic until fragrant.

- Add chicken and cook until browned on all sides.
- Add sweet potatoes, chicken broth, paprika, cayenne pepper, salt, and pepper. Bring to a boil.
- Reduce heat, cover, and simmer for 30 minutes, until the sweet potatoes are tender.
- Stir in spinach during the last 5 minutes of cooking.

Nutritional Benefits:

Sweet potatoes are high in beta-carotene, which supports the production of progesterone, essential for fertility. Chicken provides lean protein necessary for tissue repair and hormone regulation.

Nutritional Information (per serving):

- Calories: 320 kcal
- Protein: 28g
- Fat: 8g
- Carbohydrates: 40g
- Fiber: 7g
- Vitamin A: 200% RDA
- Iron: 10% RDA

Butternut Squash and Ginger Soup

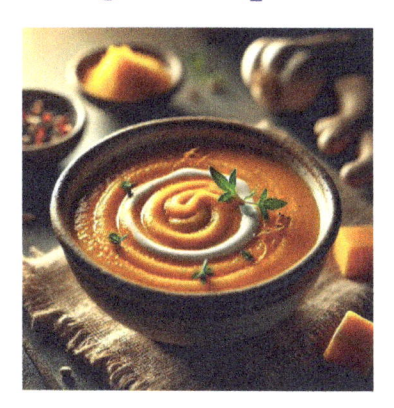

Servings: 1

Cooking Time: 30 minutes

Ingredients:

- 1 medium butternut squash, peeled and cubed
- 1 onion, chopped
- 3 garlic cloves, minced
- 1 tablespoon fresh ginger, grated
- 4 cups vegetable broth
- 1 tablespoon olive oil
- 1/2 teaspoon ground cumin
- Salt and pepper to taste

Instructions:

- Heat olive oil in a large pot over medium heat. Add onion, garlic, and ginger. Sauté until softened.

- Add cubed butternut squash, vegetable broth, cumin, salt, and pepper. Bring to a boil.
- Reduce heat and simmer for 20 minutes until the squash is tender.
- Use an immersion blender to puree the soup until smooth. Serve hot.

Nutritional Benefits:

Butternut squash is rich in vitamins A and C, both of which are important for egg quality and reducing oxidative stress. Ginger aids digestion and reduces inflammation, supporting hormonal balance.

Nutritional Information (per serving):

- Calories: 180 kcal
- Protein: 3g
- Fat: 7g
- Carbohydrates: 30g
- Fiber: 6g
- Vitamin A: 250% RDA
- Vitamin C: 40% RDA

Black Bean and Corn Chili

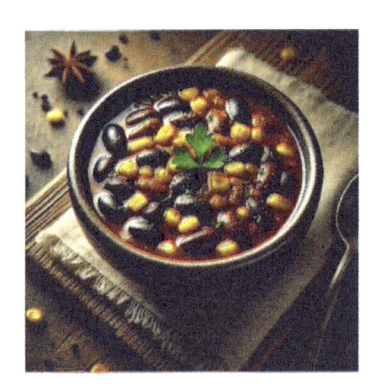

Servings: 1

Cooking Time: 40 minutes

Ingredients:

- 1 can (15 oz) black beans, drained and rinsed
- 1 can (15 oz) diced tomatoes
- 1 cup corn kernels (fresh or frozen)
- 1 onion, diced
- 2 garlic cloves, minced
- 1 tablespoon chili powder
- 1 teaspoon cumin
- 4 cups vegetable broth
- 1 tablespoon olive oil
- Salt and pepper to taste

Instructions:

- Heat olive oil in a large pot over medium heat. Sauté onion and garlic until softened.
- Add black beans, tomatoes, corn, chili powder, cumin, and vegetable broth. Stir to combine.

- Bring to a boil, reduce heat, and simmer for 30 minutes.
- Season with salt and pepper before serving.

Nutritional Benefits:

Black beans are a great source of plant-based protein and fiber, which help regulate blood sugar and support digestion—important factors in hormone balance.

Nutritional Information (per serving):

- Calories: 280 kcal
- Protein: 10g
- Fat: 6g
- Carbohydrates: 45g
- Fiber: 12g
- Iron: 15% RDA
- Folate: 35% RDA

Carrot and Red Lentil Soup

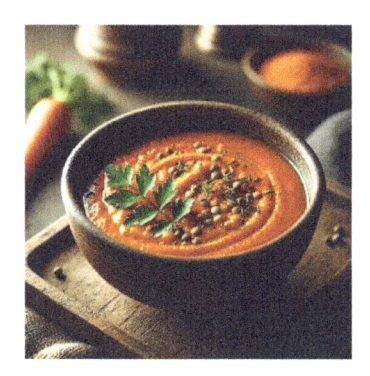

Servings: 1

Cooking Time: 30 minutes

Ingredients:

- 1 cup red lentils, rinsed
- 4 carrots, peeled and diced
- 1 onion, chopped
- 2 garlic cloves, minced
- 4 cups vegetable broth
- 1 tablespoon olive oil
- 1 teaspoon cumin
- 1/2 teaspoon turmeric
- Salt and pepper to taste

Instructions:

- Heat olive oil in a large pot over medium heat. Sauté onion, garlic, and carrots until softened.
- Add red lentils, vegetable broth, cumin, turmeric, salt, and pepper. Bring to a boil.
- Reduce heat and simmer for 20 minutes, until lentils are tender.
- Blend with an immersion blender until smooth and creamy. Serve hot.

Nutritional Benefits:

Carrots provide beta-carotene, which supports the production of hormones like progesterone. Red lentils offer fiber and protein, essential for maintaining stable blood sugar levels and energy.

Nutritional Information (per serving):

- Calories: 240 kcal
- Protein: 10g

- Fat: 6g
- Carbohydrates: 38g
- Fiber: 12g
- Vitamin A: 300% RDA
- Iron: 15% RDA

Spinach and White Bean Soup

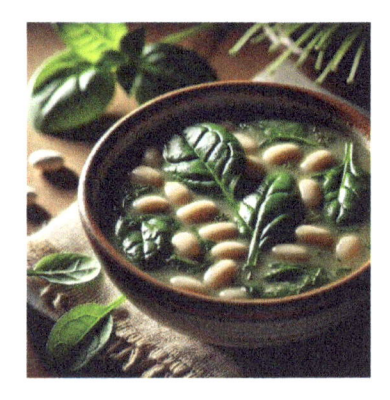

Servings: 1

Cooking Time: 25 minutes

Ingredients:

- 1 can (15 oz) white beans, drained and rinsed
- 4 cups fresh spinach
- 1 onion, diced
- 2 garlic cloves, minced
- 4 cups vegetable broth
- 1 tablespoon olive oil
- 1 teaspoon thyme
- Salt and pepper to taste

Instructions:

- Heat olive oil in a large pot over medium heat. Sauté onion and garlic until softened.
- Add white beans, spinach, vegetable broth, thyme, salt, and pepper. Bring to a boil.
- Reduce heat and simmer for 10 minutes, until spinach is wilted and tender.
- Serve hot with a drizzle of olive oil on top.

Nutritional Benefits:

Spinach is high in folate and iron, supporting reproductive health and red blood cell production. White beans provide plant-based protein and fiber, which help stabilize blood sugar.

Nutritional Information (per serving):

- Calories: 210 kcal
- Protein: 12g
- Fat: 6g
- Carbohydrates: 28g
- Fiber: 8g
- Folate: 50% RDA
- Iron: 25% RDA

Thai Coconut Chicken Soup

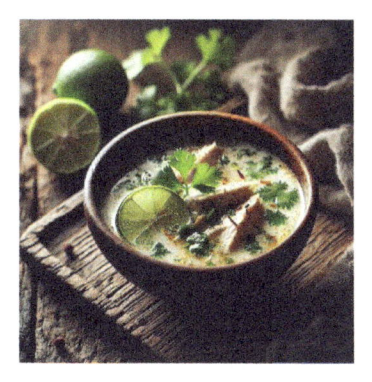

Servings: 1

Cooking Time: 30 minutes

Ingredients:

- 2 chicken breasts, thinly sliced
- 1 can (14 oz) coconut milk
- 4 cups chicken broth
- 1 tablespoon fresh ginger, grated
- 1 tablespoon fish sauce
- 1 cup mushrooms, sliced
- 1 cup baby spinach
- 1 tablespoon olive oil
- 1 tablespoon lime juice
- Salt and pepper to taste

Instructions:

- Heat olive oil in a large pot over medium heat. Sauté ginger and mushrooms until softened.
- Add chicken slices and cook until no longer pink.
- Stir in coconut milk, chicken broth, fish sauce, lime juice, and spinach. Simmer for 10 minutes, until spinach is wilted.
- Season with salt and pepper and serve hot.

Nutritional Benefits:

Coconut milk provides healthy fats that support hormone production, while chicken offers lean protein. Spinach and ginger add antioxidants and anti-inflammatory benefits, promoting hormonal balance.

Nutritional Information (per serving):

- Calories: 320 kcal
- Protein: 25g
- Fat: 20g
- Carbohydrates: 12g
- Fiber: 3g
- Iron: 15% RDA
- Vitamin C: 20% RDA

Tomato and Basil Soup

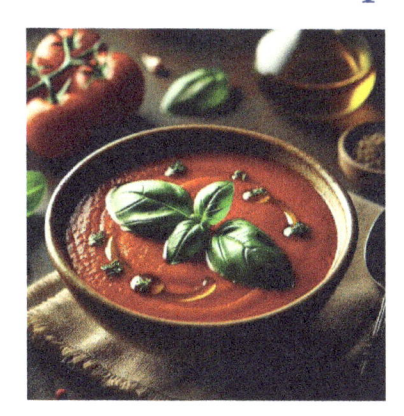

Servings: 1

Cooking Time: 25 minutes

Ingredients:

- 4 large tomatoes, chopped
- 1 onion, diced
- 3 garlic cloves, minced
- 4 cups vegetable broth
- 1/4 cup fresh basil leaves, chopped
- 1 tablespoon olive oil
- Salt and pepper to taste

Instructions:

- Heat olive oil in a pot over medium heat. Sauté onion and garlic until fragrant.
- Add chopped tomatoes, vegetable broth, salt, and pepper. Bring to a boil, then reduce heat and simmer for 20 minutes.
- Use an immersion blender to puree the soup until smooth.
- Stir in fresh basil and serve.

Nutritional Benefits:

Tomatoes are rich in lycopene, an antioxidant that supports reproductive health by reducing oxidative stress. Basil adds anti-inflammatory properties, further supporting overall hormonal balance.

Nutritional Information (per serving):

- Calories: 180 kcal
- Protein: 4g
- Fat: 6g
- Carbohydrates: 28g
- Fiber: 6g
- Vitamin C: 40% RDA
- Iron: 10% RDA

Moroccan Chickpea Stew

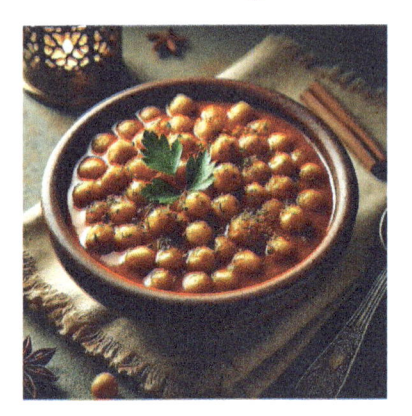

Servings: 1

Cooking Time: 40 minutes

Ingredients:

- 1 can (15 oz) chickpeas, drained and rinsed
- 1 onion, diced
- 2 carrots, sliced
- 2 garlic cloves, minced
- 1 tablespoon tomato paste
- 4 cups vegetable broth
- 1 teaspoon ground cumin
- 1 teaspoon paprika
- 1/2 teaspoon cinnamon
- 1 tablespoon olive oil
- Salt and pepper to taste

Instructions:

- Heat olive oil in a large pot over medium heat. Sauté onion, carrots, and garlic until softened.
- Stir in tomato paste, cumin, paprika, and cinnamon. Cook for 2 minutes.
- Add chickpeas and vegetable broth. Simmer for 30 minutes, until the flavors are combined.
- Season with salt and pepper before serving.

Nutritional Benefits:

Chickpeas provide protein and fiber, helping to stabilize blood sugar and improve digestion. Cinnamon has anti-inflammatory properties and supports insulin sensitivity, benefiting reproductive health.

Nutritional Information (per serving):

- Calories: 280 kcal
- Protein: 10g
- Fat: 8g
- Carbohydrates: 40g
- Fiber: 10g
- Iron: 15% RDA
- Folate: 20% RDA

Kale and Quinoa Soup

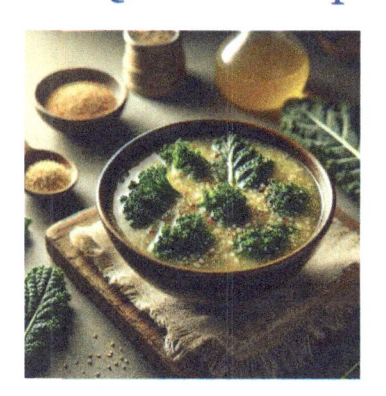

Servings: 1

Cooking Time: 30 minutes

Ingredients:

- 1 cup cooked quinoa
- 4 cups fresh kale, chopped
- 1 onion, diced
- 2 garlic cloves, minced
- 4 cups vegetable broth
- 1 tablespoon olive oil
- 1 teaspoon thyme
- Salt and pepper to taste

Instructions:

- Heat olive oil in a pot over medium heat. Sauté onion and garlic until softened.
- Add vegetable broth, thyme, kale, and quinoa. Bring to a boil.
- Reduce heat and simmer for 20 minutes.
- Season with salt and pepper, and serve hot.

Nutritional Benefits:

Kale is packed with vitamins A and C, which support egg health and boost the immune system. Quinoa is a complete protein, offering all essential amino acids needed for hormone production.

Nutritional Information (per serving):

- Calories: 220 kcal
- Protein: 8g
- Fat: 7g
- Carbohydrates: 34g
- Fiber: 7g
- Vitamin A: 150% RDA
- Iron: 20% RDA

CHAPTER 7

4-Week Meal Plan for IVF Mothers

Week 1

Day 1

Breakfast: Chia Seed and Almond Butter Smoothie Bowl

Lunch: Quinoa and Avocado Salad with Lemon Tahini Dressing

Dinner: Baked Salmon with Asparagus and Quinoa

Snack: Greek Yogurt with Pumpkin Seeds and Berries

Day 2

Breakfast: Avocado and Egg Toast

Lunch: Grilled Chicken and Kale Salad with Pumpkin Seeds

Dinner: Lentil and Sweet Potato Curry

Snack: Almond and Chia Seed Energy Bites

Day 3

Breakfast: Spinach and Feta Omelet

Lunch: Roasted Vegetable and Farro Bowl

Dinner: Cod with Spinach and White Beans

Snack: Apple Slices with Almond Butter

Day 4

Breakfast: Overnight Oats with Flaxseeds and Berries

Lunch: Beet and Goat Cheese Salad with Walnuts

Dinner: Turkey and Zucchini Meatballs with Tomato Sauce

Snack: Roasted Chickpeas with Spices

Day 5

Breakfast: Quinoa Breakfast Bowl with Almonds and Apples

Lunch: Grilled Salmon and Quinoa Salad with Lemon Vinaigrette

Dinner: Eggplant and Chickpea Stew

Snack: Hard-Boiled Eggs with Avocado

Day 6

Breakfast: Chia Pudding with Coconut and Mango

Lunch: Lentil and Spinach Soup

Dinner: Grilled Chicken with Roasted Vegetables

Snack: Celery Sticks with Hummus

Day 7

Breakfast: Greek Yogurt with Honey and Walnuts

Lunch: Turkey and Zucchini Meatballs with Tomato Sauce

Dinner: Baked Salmon with Asparagus and Quinoa

Snack: Banana and Peanut Butter Smoothie

Week 2

Day 1

Breakfast: Spinach and Feta Omelette

Lunch: Quinoa and Avocado Salad with Lemon Tahini Dressing

Dinner: Grilled Chicken with Roasted Vegetables

Snack: Greek Yogurt with Pumpkin Seeds and Berries

Day 2

Breakfast: Chia Pudding with Coconut and Mango

Lunch: Lentil and Spinach Soup

Dinner: Cod with Spinach and White Beans

Snack: Almond and Chia Seed Energy Bites

Day 3

Breakfast: Overnight Oats with Flaxseeds and Berries

Lunch: Roasted Vegetable and Farro Bowl

Dinner: Baked Salmon with Asparagus and Quinoa

Snack: Apple Slices with Almond Butter

Day 4

Breakfast: Avocado and Egg Toast

Lunch: Beet and Goat Cheese Salad with Walnuts

Dinner: Lentil and Sweet Potato Curry

Snack: Hard-Boiled Eggs with Avocado

Day 5

Breakfast: Quinoa Breakfast Bowl with Almonds and Apples

Lunch: Grilled Chicken and Kale Salad with Pumpkin Seeds

Dinner: Eggplant and Chickpea Stew

Snack: Roasted Chickpeas with Spices

Day 6

Breakfast: Chia Seed and Almond Butter Smoothie Bowl

Lunch: Grilled Salmon and Quinoa Salad with Lemon Vinaigrette

Dinner: Turkey and Zucchini Meatballs with Tomato Sauce

Snack: Celery Sticks with Hummus

Day 7

Breakfast: Spinach and Feta Omelet

Lunch: Lentil and Spinach Soup

Dinner: Cod with Spinach and White Beans

Snack: Greek Yogurt with Honey and Walnuts

Week 3

Day 1

Breakfast: Chia Pudding with Coconut and Mango

Lunch: Grilled Chicken and Kale Salad with Pumpkin Seeds

Dinner: Baked Salmon with Asparagus and Quinoa

Snack: Greek Yogurt with Honey and Walnuts

Day 2

Breakfast: Overnight Oats with Flaxseeds and Berries

Lunch: Beet and Goat Cheese Salad with Walnuts

Dinner: Lentil and Sweet Potato Curry

Snack: Hard-Boiled Eggs with Avocado

Day 3

Breakfast: Quinoa Breakfast Bowl with Almonds and Apples

Lunch: Roasted Vegetable and Farro Bowl

Dinner: Grilled Chicken with Roasted Vegetables

Snack: Apple Slices with Almond Butter

Day 4

Breakfast: Spinach and Feta Omelet

Lunch: Lentil and Spinach Soup

Dinner: Cod with Spinach and White Beans

Snack: Roasted Chickpeas with Spices

Day 5

Breakfast: Avocado and Egg Toast

Lunch: Grilled Salmon and Quinoa Salad with Lemon Vinaigrette

Dinner: Eggplant and Chickpea Stew

Snack: Celery Sticks with Hummus

Day 6

Breakfast: Chia Seed and Almond Butter Smoothie Bowl

Lunch: Turkey and Zucchini Meatballs with Tomato Sauce

Dinner: Lentil and Sweet Potato Curry

Snack: Greek Yogurt with Pumpkin Seeds and Berries

Day 7

Breakfast: Greek Yogurt with Honey and Walnuts

Lunch: Grilled Chicken and Kale Salad with Pumpkin Seeds

Dinner: Baked Salmon with Asparagus and Quinoa

Snack: Banana and Peanut Butter Smoothie

Week 4

Day 1

Breakfast: Quinoa Breakfast Bowl with Almonds and Apples

Lunch: Beet and Goat Cheese Salad with Walnuts

Dinner: Lentil and Sweet Potato Curry

Snack: Roasted Chickpeas with Spices

Day 2

Breakfast: Avocado and Egg Toast

Lunch: Grilled Chicken and Kale Salad with Pumpkin Seeds

Dinner: Cod with Spinach and White Beans

Snack: Greek Yogurt with Honey and Walnuts

Day 3

Breakfast: Chia Pudding with Coconut and Mango

Lunch: Grilled Salmon and Quinoa Salad with Lemon Vinaigrette

Dinner: Eggplant and Chickpea Stew

Snack: Celery Sticks with Hummus

Day 4

Breakfast: Spinach and Feta omelet

Lunch: Roasted Vegetable and Farro Bowl

Dinner: Lentil and Sweet Potato Curry

Snack: Almond and Chia Seed Energy Bites

Day 5

Breakfast: Overnight Oats with Flaxseeds and Berries

Lunch: Lentil and Spinach Soup

Dinner: Grilled Chicken with Roasted Vegetables

Snack: Apple Slices with Almond Butter

Day 6

Breakfast: Chia Seed and Almond Butter Smoothie Bowl

Lunch: Beet and Goat Cheese Salad with Walnuts

Dinner: Baked Salmon with Asparagus and Quinoa

Snack: Greek Yogurt with Pumpkin Seeds and Berries

Day 7

Breakfast: Quinoa Breakfast Bowl with Almonds and Apples

Lunch: Grilled Salmon and Quinoa Salad with Lemon Vinaigrette

Dinner: Cod with Spinach and White Beans

Snack: Hard-Boiled Eggs with Avocado

SHOPPING LIST

Fruits:
- Bananas
- Apples
- Avocados
- Berries (blueberries, raspberries, strawberries)
- Lemon
- Mango
- Pineapple
- Mixed fresh or frozen berries
- Sweet potatoes
- Tomatoes
- Zucchini
- Cucumbers

Vegetables:
- Spinach
- Kale
- Carrots
- Celery
- Red bell pepper
- Onions
- Garlic cloves
- Cherry tomatoes
- Butternut squash
- Broccoli
- Brussels sprouts
- Mushrooms
- Asparagus
- Eggplant
- Mixed greens (e.g., arugula, spinach)
- Parsley
- Basil

Grains:
- Whole-grain or sprouted bread
- Quinoa
- Rolled oats
- Almond flour
- Farro
- Whole-grain tortillas
- Corn kernels

Proteins:
- Eggs (organic if possible)
- Chicken breasts and thighs
- Salmon
- Shrimp
- Ground turkey
- Tofu (firm)
- Black beans
- White beans
- Lentils (red, dried, and green)
- Chickpeas (canned or dried)

Dairy or Dairy Alternatives:
- Greek yogurt (or dairy-free alternative)

- Cottage cheese (or dairy-free alternative)
- Feta cheese

Nuts & Seeds:

- Almond butter
- Slivered almonds
- Walnuts
- Chia seeds
- Flaxseeds
- Pumpkin seeds
- Cashews

Condiments & Oils:

- Olive oil
- Coconut oil
- Sesame oil
- Soy sauce or tamari (for gluten-free)
- Tahini
- Honey or maple syrup
- Dark chocolate chips (optional)
- Balsamic vinegar
- Fish sauce
- Vanilla extract

Spices & Seasonings:

- Salt and pepper
- Paprika (regular and smoked)
- Cumin
- Cinnamon
- Turmeric
- Dried oregano
- Fresh ginger
- Red pepper flakes
- Thyme
- Rosemary

Special Ingredients:

- Chia seeds
- Coconut milk (unsweetened)
- Dark chocolate (70% cacao or higher)

Made in United States
North Haven, CT
10 January 2025